MEDITATION FOR BEGINNERS

MEDITATION THE KEY TO HAPPINESS

100 Meditations for Healing, Success, and Peace

ARI BOND

Table of Contents

PART I

Chapter 1: Health Benefits of Decluttering

The idea of clutter has many different meanings. In its simplest terms, it explains the physical things that provide no real meaning, but just fill space. These things can be anything from a pile of old newspapers in your home, to clothes that no longer fit, or something that just no longer serves a purpose. While these physical objects are truly just "things" that take up space in your home, they also take up space in your mind.

Right now, you are likely sitting at home or at work reading this book. Take a look around. Is your space clean and clutter-free, or are there a bunch of little things all around you? More importantly, do all of those little things actually serve a purpose, or are you not really sure why they are there?

If you aren't sure why you have so many things, it is time to seriously consider decluttering your space. You see, stuff isn't just stuff, it develops an emotional connection within you. A cluttered home indicates a cluttered mind, and a cluttered home also causes a disorganized mind. This is a two-way street. The clutter probably built up because of distraction within your brain.

Many of us don't feel the need to save a pile of junk mail, yet there it may sit on the kitchen counter for weeks. A clear, undistracted mind would have the capability to quickly and systematically sort through that mail, and discard the unimportant things. Instead, the mind thinks of ten other things at once, and going through the mail becomes a daunting task. When you feel distracted, it is easy to let the little things go, which leads to unneeded things cluttering your life.

Unfortunately, this is a vicious circle. Yes, your mind was working on ten different projects before the mail came, but by not getting through the mail pile, you have inadvertently created the eleventh, furthering your mind from being free.

The "stuff" is both the cause and effect of a cluttered mind, and the only way to break that cycle is to decrease the clutter.

Not only are those excess things causing a cluttered mind, they also hold emotional baggage. Think about that pair of jeans sitting in your closet. They were a size too small when you bought them, but at that time, you promised yourself that you would lose a few pounds and they would fit. Several years later, they still sit there, in the bag you brought them home in, with the tags still on. They are no longer just a pair of pants, they are a sign of failure. You failed to reach your weight loss goal, and those pants are a daily reminder of your shortcomings. Getting dressed in the morning should not come with a dose of negativity.

Any type of object could hold negative thoughts and feelings, and we must recognize these things and remove them from our lives. The simple act of removing something that evokes bad feelings or memories can have a tremendous effect on our mental health and emotional state. Decluttering can be a very emotional process for some due to these connections. For example, after losing a loved one, it is common for mourners to keep rooms or other living spaces exactly as the deceased left it. The things inside that room become a sort of shrine to the departed, and instead of being inanimate objects, become an emotional crutch. For some, it may be necessary to seek help from a therapist to deal with the emotional connection before getting rid of the things.

From an artistic standpoint, a mess of clutter is unappealing to the eye. In art, it is the artists' responsibility to draw the eye in at a focal point, and let the eye flow over the picture and back to the focal point in a swift, easy motion. When someone doesn't know where to look, the brain gets confused and begins to use more energy searching for a focal point. The same is true with the spaces we inhabit. If your bedroom has clothes all over the floor, and the bedsheets and blankets crumpled into a ball, your eyes see chaos and expend more energy trying to make sense of it. You are draining your own emotional energy by living in this environment. When was the last time you saw a cluttered room on the front page of a home improvement magazine?

Decluttering gives your mind more time to focus on important things. By removing menial thoughts of cleaning up the house, it leaves more room for focusing on tasks at work, or simply becoming more present in your life. Many people find that decluttering actually enhances their performance at work. As their brains become less distracted, they have more power to focus on projects at work, and their energy and mental focus are greatly improved.

This can translate to other areas of life, like being mentally present when hanging out with friends, spouses, and kids, leading to more meaningful and satisfying relationships. Studies prove that having these types of relationships in your life is a direct indicator of happiness and improved mental status.

Many professional organizers can attest to improvements of their clients' mental as well as physical health. The immediate decrease in stress by changing the living environment boosts the mood and energy, lowers blood pressure and promotes health and weight loss, likely due from overall decreases in stress. In extreme cases, like hoarding, excess clutter gathers dust and critters that live in the mess. This could be a health hazard, creating breathing problems and increases the risk of fire.

Take another look around. What is the current state of your surroundings? If you are feeling overwhelmed by the chaos of clutter around you, or even think that some minor improvements can be made, go ahead and get started. Make a commitment to reduce your clutter for the sake of your physical health and well-being.

Chapter 2: Joys Of Simple Living

Over the past decade or so, our culture has taken a drastic

turn. Earlier decades played up the need for having extravagant things. Buying new cars, the best new video games, and fancy new clothes every season was the norm, and if you wanted to have any sort of popular status, this is what you did.

Besides the problems in funding behind these habits, we found that having all of this "stuff" really served no emotional purpose. Things don't make you truly happy, and buying a new pair of shoes every time things get tough causes you to avoid solving the problem. As this fact came to light, many people started to shy away from physical things and were drawn more to meaningful relationships and memorable experiences as a way to find happiness in life. While there are still many stragglers on this earth, studies have shown that people who have less "stuff" are generally happier in life. So, there is only one reasonable conclusion; get rid of your clutter!

The things in your home should only be those that bring you joy or serve a regular purpose. Hanging on to other things that you may use someday, like those jeans that are two sizes too small, really serves no purpose. It is time to retrain your brain to look at your things as the inanimate objects that they are. Things only have meaning because we cause them to. The baseball you brought home from a game isn't special, it is the memory of going to that game with your family. Hold on to the memory (and a few pictures), but remember that the baseball is just a baseball.

Take it one step further. That baseball could be used to create more great memories. If you or your kids aren't interested in playing with it, give it to the kids down the block. Take note when you see them outside playing, knowing that you brought them a little bit of joy. That is worth much more than leather and string.

Most importantly, get rid of things that trigger bad memories. This can be a tough thing, especially if you feel that keeping certain items are a replacement for something you have lost. Unfortunately, we all lost people, or favorite pets over the course of our lives. Let's say your dog died, and you decide to hold on to their collar. That collar may bring back memories of great times with your dog, but may also make you sad that they're gone. While it's okay to miss them, that collar is not required to have those memories. If you were to take a souvenir from every memory you ever had, your house would be filled to the brim.

If you feel ready, donate the collar to another dog. Whether that means adopting a new dog or giving it to a friend, give that collar good use and honor your fallen friend by letting her live on. If you're not ready to take that step, go ahead and keep it. That's right, keep it. Having certain things of meaning in your home is important as well. But maybe get rid of the old dog toys as a compromise. Once you are ready to let go, make that choice.

Simple living isn't just limited to the physical things in life, it is also the processes in which we live our daily life. The majority of people would say they hit the ground running as soon as the alarm goes off. They are pulled in different directions, trying to pack lunches and get kids on the bus, satisfying the needs of others at work, then going to obligatory meetings like PTA, or community council meetings. Remember that events in your calendar are "things" too. They are things that are getting in the way of your happiness. If you truly enjoy these things, go ahead and keep them in your schedule. If you hate extracurricular meetings after work, take a step back.

Life is meant to be lived in a satisfying way. If you feel that your current course of activities is simply to please others, it is time to reevaluate your priorities. Make happiness a priority too. There will be things you have to do, but you don't have to do those things all the time. Start scheduling in fun activities instead of doing them only when there is extra time.

Take a look at your calendar. Change the color of all work events to blue, or a color of choice. Next, make obligatory meetings, like book club, yellow. Finally, make fun outings pink. What does your calendar look like? Is it a sea of blue and yellow, or a colorful patchwork of work and fun?

As you plan next week, mark out some time for doing a workout class with a friend, catching up on reading, or any other activity that brings you joy. While we all have obligations, a life isn't worth living if that work isn't balanced out by a bit of fun. Learn how to say 'no' if a special project just doesn't seem appealing, and set some time aside for things you truly love. You won't want to get to the end of your life and realize you just worked.

Chapter 3: Clutter Overhaul

Now that you realize how important decluttering can be to your overall health, it's time to make a plan. How you will carry out that plan will really depend on the level of clutter in your home. For the sake of covering everyone, let's say you have developed quite a bit of clutter, in which only about half of the things in your home have any use to you. This might be you if every stable surface in your home is loaded with things, you constantly trip over stuff, or if you have entire rooms you have not entered in years, due to a number of things that have accumulated.

While it may seem overwhelming, the best thing to do is rip off the bandage and just get started. Clear your schedule for an entire weekend, or plan to take a couple of days off from work, to spend cleaning and organizing. Set up a schedule for yourself if that makes it seem a little less overwhelming. While there is something to be said for making changes a little bit at a time, sometimes it's easier to get these things done in one big session, rather than dragging out the process.

If you feel that a big cleanout is not feasible, do what you can, and at least commit to a daily 5 minute declutter, which will be discussed in the last chapter.

Start with the most frequently used room in the house. Dedicate your time to completing this one room before moving on. Look at it and make a mental checklist of the things that need to be done, then go ahead and tackle it.

Before you begin, make sure you have a plan to get rid of these things. Simply moving them to other rooms, or bagging it all up to sit on the porch, have a clear plan for things to move to other locations besides your home. This can mean a few things. You can either bite the bullet and throw things away, like true garbage, sell items of value, like collectibles you no longer care about or donate gently used items to others. While it is best to recycle what you can, sometimes figuring out the minute details of getting that done can be overwhelming. Try to figure it out ahead of time so you don't get discouraged while you clean.

Call up a local shelter or charity to let them know you have children's toys, or old clothing, or anything else that might be helpful. This serves as a place to dispense of old items, and getting others involved makes you committed to your cleanout. This is especially important if you either do have things of great value, like collectibles you no longer want, or useful things that you will have a hard time throwing in the trash.

Take regular breaks, drinking water and eating, to keep up your strength and willpower. One of the reasons we avoid overhauls like this is because it is mentally and physically draining. It can be emotionally equivalent to packing all of your things and moving. Just exhausting. Take breaks, revisit why you are doing this to begin with, and keep up the motivation.

If you have a hard time letting things go, develop a system to get through it. For example, if you feel that everything is sentimental, like the same level as the dog collar, a simple set of rules can help you distinguish between truly sentimental and borderline hoarding tendencies.

Rules for decluttering:

Rule #1: If you haven't used an item in over 6 months, it's time to let go.

Rule #2: If you didn't know you had an item, and it serves no purpose to better your life, let it go.

Rule #3: If an item brings back negative memories or emotions, let go.

Don't be afraid to ask for help. Just like moving, decluttering may be something your friends or family will dread helping with. But, as friends and family do, they can recognize a plea for help and would like to help you improve your life. Ask for a bit of help, and make sure to keep the mood light and airy as you work. Commiserating about all of the things still left to do will only bring the process down. Decluttering is about freeing yourself, so keep the tone that way.

Certain cases of clutter require a bit more help and don't be afraid to ask. Some of you reading this may have a legitimate problem with hoarding. There has been a lot of light shed on this problem in recent years, as TV programs have been dedicated to this subject. While the people on those shows are fascinating cases, the underlying psychological issues that are associated with this habit are apparent.

Just like a substance abuse or overeating problem, hoarding tendencies are a real, diagnosable problem that can be treated with therapy and with the help of a professional organizer. To generalize, people who hoard either never learned proper housekeeping habits, or use their hoarding as a coping mechanism for past or current trauma, like the death of a loved one, or abuse, much like someone with a drug problem would. It is important not to make light of people who have this type of problem. Hoarding is an addiction too.

Good did come from the spotlight, however. Therapy services and professional organizing and cleanup services specialize in managing hoards, and the media showed how the recovery process worked so that people with no idea where to start fixing their problem had a guide to help them. There is nothing worse than recognizing you have a problem, but not knowing how to fix it. Seek the help of a therapist if you feel there are underlying issues attached to your collecting and saving tendencies. At least, they will help you get to the root of the problem to stop the habit, but they also will likely have ideas to help you clean up, giving references to local companies. Seeking out help will probably be the most difficult, but most beneficial step in the healing process.

No matter your level of decluttering, use these rules to help get started. As you make decisions to get rid of things, your mind will start to clear and you will have the confidence to complete your project and better your life. If you begin to feel overwhelmed, think about how nice your home will look, and how clear your thoughts will be when you're done!

Chapter 4: The 5 Minute Daily Declutter

Five minutes isn't long. It takes about five minutes to brew a pot of coffee, go outside and get the mail, or even brush your teeth. Why not devote just five minutes a day to decluttering your home, for the sake of your health?

If you completed an entire decluttering overhaul, as outlined in Chapter 3, a five minute declutter should be just about all you need to maintain your clutter-free home. After all, once you start from scratch, you should no longer have piles of things to put away, just what is left over from the day.

The time of day in which you complete this five minutes is up to you, but many people benefit from doing this as part of their morning routine. If you leave it for the end of the day, you will likely be tired and mentally drained. Purposefully picking things up and putting them where they belong can sometimes take a bit of thought, which you will likely have more energy for first thing in the morning.

So today, after you finish reading this book, set a timer for five minutes. Use the timer on your phone or microwave. Begin picking up things that don't belong where they are, like clothes on the floor, junk mail sitting on the counter, anything that is out of place. Likely, you will find yourself getting impatient with your own daily habits. In five minutes a day, you will begin to realize just how much chaos you accumulate in one day. Why couldn't you have put the clothes in the laundry basket across the room once you took them off? Why did you wait until the next day to put them in there?

As you begin to notice these annoying self-habits, you will likely correct them, leading to less clutter in the first place. Your five minutes will become more and more productive, as less time will be needed for the things you should have done, to begin with.

It is important to do one item at a time during your five minutes. Pick up the clothes and either fold and put them away, or throw them in the laundry basket. Put the book you finished back on the shelf, instead of letting it sit on the coffee table. Purposefully put each item where it belongs, don't just stick it on an already-overflowing shelf. No, you won't go back to it later, do it now.

Make a point to start in a different room each day. Constantly starting in the kitchen, then living room, then bedroom, means that the dining room never gets any attention. Each day, start in the room that needs the most attention or has had the most neglect.

If you didn't participate in a full home overhaul, your space may need a bit more work. Let's say your kitchen needs to be reorganized. Use that daily five minutes to clean out one drawer at a time, moving or getting rid of things that don't belong in that drawer, or things you simply have no use for. While it will take a lot longer to completely declutter your home with five minutes a day, if decluttering is emotionally draining for you, five minutes may be all you can handle. When you're feeling motivated, go ahead and do more, but commit yourself to at least five minutes. It will be over before you know it!

Chapter 5: Organization 101

The primary purpose for decluttering your living space is for functionality, and that starts with organization. Think about the layout of your kitchen. If you wanted to make a batch of brownies right now, can you think of where all of the ingredients are? The pan to cook it in? Like many of us, that baking pan is probably at the bottom of a stack of pans and involves a bit of finagling to get it out of its hiding place. Perhaps you don't know where your baking chocolate or flour is. The goal of the organization is for everything important to have its place so that you know where to find it. In the grand scheme of things, this will save you time, and an exorbitant amount of frustration when it comes to daily tasks.

Take this mindset to other areas of your home. Is all of your makeup stuffed in a single bag? And where is that red lipstick? These little, seemingly insignificant thoughts, on top of a hundred others, can leave you mentally drained before you even leave the house in the morning. Just thinking of it now may make you feel a bit overwhelmed. If everything had a place, and you knew where to look, everyday tasks would become just a bit easier, leaving energy for your mind to focus on more pertinent things.

Now is the time to take action. Now that you have gotten rid of a lot of things that you simply don't need, it is time to organize your daily essentials in a way that fits your needs. All of the things you need to get ready for work in the morning should be in the same place. Your clothes should be clean, folded or hung, and ready to go. Your toothpaste, deodorant, and other hygiene products should be in one place. In the kitchen, your egg pan should be clean and put away, ready for use, and as you pack your lunch, you shouldn't be digging in the back of the cabinet to find a lid for the plastic wear. All of these things add up to wasted valuable time.

Decide to organize one room at a time. It is important to focus on one space. Take the kitchen, for example. Take a few minutes to think about your normal kitchen workflow.

If you are constantly searching for a spatula or wooden spoon while you cook, make sure to store those utensils in a drawer closest to the stove. Knives and cutting boards should be relatively close to each other. Baking pans should have racks. Utilize counter space only for those things you use every single day, like a blender or toaster. If you are short on counter space, keep your work area as clutter-free as possible to avoid frustration. Everything should have a place, and you shouldn't have to move five things to do one simple task.

Next, systematically go through your closets. We all have that one closet that becomes a dumping ground. Kids closets are often filled with broken or unused toys. Likely, the things they like most are out in their bedroom, so the closet is a great place to start when thinning the junk. First, get rid of anything broken. Don't fall for the practical side of your brain when it says, "I can fix that!". If you do not actively fix that within a few minutes, it will just continue to sit in the closet. Get rid of it!

Clothes in an adult closet are the same as toys. If there are clothes you never wear, that don't fit, or simply aren't your style, why do you have them? Since clothes are expensive, it can be hard to let go. Do your best to give away clothes that are still in good shape. Give things to friends, sell them at a consignment shop, or donate them to charity. For old clothes with holes and stains, throw them out, or throw them in the rag pile in the garage. They will still be good for dusting the house or checking the oil in your car. Just don't get carried away. Save a few good ones and discard the rest.

No home is complete without a junk drawer. This is a place where all of the little things that just don't fit in go. Store things like batteries, tape, thumbtacks, glue and other small items in your junk drawer. You may think this isn't organized, but it truly is. Everything has its place, and if it doesn't it's placed is the junk drawer. In the event you need one of these random items, you will know exactly where to look. Over time, your junk drawer will upgrade to a magic junk drawer, producing just the right item when you need it most!

When it comes to organization and decluttering, it is best to use what you already have, and avoid buying more things to keep in your home. Use old baskets or bags for storage. Reorganize dressers and bureaus to fit more, and utilize space under the bed.

In some cases, it will be necessary to buy organizational products. A full closet organizer system probably isn't required for most people, but a pack of new hangers and a couple of baskets can turn a closet into a more organized, functional space. Purchase large, flat containers to store off-season clothes under the bed, or a filing cabinet to keep your important papers organized. Just don't go overboard, as you will end up with more junk! Think function.

PART II

CHAPTER ONE

A WARNING

Everybody is different, making every habit different. That means that all these tips coming up are subjective. It's not something that will work for everybody. Another thing you need to be aware of is that your habit could be something more. I'm going to go over this possible problem quickly. Keep in mind this is not to cure or diagnose you with anything. If you think you may have a psychological disorder, as opposed to a bad habit, please seek medical attention.

For your information, a habit is defined as a settled or regular tendency or practice; especially one that is hard to give up.

OCD, obsessive compulsive disorder, can be confused as a habit. OCD can fall into four main categories;

- checking

- contamination/mental contamination

- hoarding

- ruminations/intrusive thoughts

OCD is diagnosed by when obsessions and compulsions:

- Consume excessive amounts of time

- Causes significant distress

- Interferes with daily functions

Your habit, itself, could be OCD, or your inability to break the habit, could be caused by OCD. An example of OCD being the habit would be hoarding. An example of OCD interfering your ability to break a habit would be intrusive thoughts. Now, when breaking a habit you will have intrusive thoughts, but they should just come and go. If your intrusive thoughts are constant and interfere with your life, then OCD could be a factor.

Other psychological disorders that could be confused with a habit are, eating disorders. Anorexia nervosa and bulimia nervosa are common eating disorders where people end up starving themselves or binging and purging. A lesser known eating disorder, which is the one most likely to be confused as a habit, is a binge-eating disorder.

With binge-eating disorder, people lose control of their eating habits. Unlike with bulimia nervosa, periods of binges are not followed by purging, which is why most people with binge-eating disorder are overweight. It is the top eating disorder in the US. Symptoms of binge-eating disorder are:

- Eating an unusually large amount of food in a specific amount of time

- Eating even when you're full or not hungry

- Eating fast during binge episodes

- Eating until you are uncomfortably full

- Eating alone or in secret to avoid embarrassment

- Feeling distressed, ashamed, or guilty when not eating

- Frequent dieting, possibly without weight loss

Chances are everybody can say that they have experienced one or more of these symptoms. For example, most holidays' people will over eat. That does not mean you have binge-eating disorder. Keep in mind disorders interrupt your everyday life, and happen constantly. If you just overeat when watching TV, or when you're bored, then you probably don't have a disorder. If you are concerned that you might, then please seek medical advice.

Make sure that if you think you have a disorder to see your doctor make sure. It's better to believe you have a disease than go around with an undiagnosed disorder. I want to make sure that you can live the life you deserve and making sure that your habit isn't something more serious is important.

CHAPTER TWO

A HISTORY OF HABITS

Imagine this; your alarm goes off. You slide out of bed and slump your way to the bathroom. You do your business and then hop in the shower. Once finished you brush your teeth before you get dressed. Once dressed you head to the kitchen to have your coffee and breakfast. Now, what just happened? You were on complete autopilot. You are so used to doing the same thing every morning you don't have to think about it. That is what a habit is.

Human beings are creatures of habit. We get into a routine, and we stick to it. Then it becomes a struggle to change.

Chances are your habits are caused by stress or boredom. You start doing things to distract your brain from the stress or boredom, giving you brain a brief moment of utopia.

Stress and boredom aren't just triggers for certain habits. They're triggers for most habits. Whether you have a problem with eating, smoking, biting your nails, or spending mindless hours on the computer, whatever it may be you're using the habit to suppress those emotions. There is a chance that a deeper issue causes the stress or boredom that is being felt.

Ask yourself, is there a belief or a reason you're holding onto this habit?

The key to overcoming a habit is to figure out what is causing it. Did something happen when you were younger? Do you believe something bad is going to happen if you stop?

That's why there is no one solution. Take the habit of smoking. According to the World Health Organization, more than one billion people smoke. Most of those people are smoking for different reasons. Some may smoke because they saw their parents smoke, or their friends. They may have started smoking as a way to cope with stress.

A Loop

Every habit begins with a psychological pattern. The habit loop is a three-part process. It begins with a trigger. The trigger tells you brain to go into automatic mode and let a behavior happen. The second part is the routine which is the actual habit itself. The last part is the reward. The reward is something your brain likes and helps it remember the loop in the future.

According to neuroscientists, habit-making behaviors are controlled in the basal ganglia. The basal ganglia are also the area of the brain that controls emotions, memories, and patterns. As stated above, a habit is a pattern.

Decisions are controlled in the prefrontal cortex. A habit starts as a behavior or decision, but the more you do it, the less the brain works. The decision-making part of your brain goes to sleep. That's what makes multitasking possible.

Good habits are programmed the same as bad habits are. A good habit, such as brushing your teeth, gets programmed by repetition just like smoking. Or learning to parallel park works the same as overeating.

The fact that they work the same is a good thing. That makes it easier for you to retrain your brain.

Problems

There are going to be problems when trying to break a habit, especially if your habit involves any stimulant. At that point, you're not just trying to stop the habit, but also working through the detox symptoms. For example, nicotine, via tobacco, is one of the most heavily consumed drugs in the world. In Australia, smoking is one of the biggest causes of, preventable, death, killing about 15,000 people per year. It's also one of the hardest to quit. Withdrawal from nicotine can cause insomnia, irritability, anxiety, and difficulty concentrating.

Slip-ups are inevitable, but if you're working to break a habit that involves any stimulating drug, it's going to be a lot harder. This could include smoking, drinking, even coffee. Keep this in the back of your mind so that you are prepared.

CHAPTER THREE

A HABITS HABITAT

Necessarily true. You can control your habits, but your environment plays a huge part of what you do on a daily basis. One of your brain's primary functions is to find and use patterns as shortcuts to process the information we're presented with on a daily basis.

In a study conducted on habits vs. intentions, researchers found that students that switched Universities were more likely to change their daily habits. Those habits were easier to change than they were for the control group because they weren't exposed to familiar daily cues. This can be seen in every bad habit that somebody has.

Eating Habits

Have you ever been driving home from work, not thinking about food, when you see your favorite fast food joint, and suddenly your start craving a cheeseburger? It's not your fault. Everybody experiences moments like that.

Our food environment is broken down into two categories; the atmosphere we encounter when eating, and how food is portioned. The cues vary from what's being eaten, its packaging or utensil size, and the amount of food. Think about when you eat out. You will undoubtedly receive a huge plate of food. You don't think you can eat it all, but then you end up cleaning your plate. Seeing an empty plate signals satiety in our brains.

Maybe eating at home will help you avoid these triggers. Not so fast. Home plate sizes have increased 22% over the last century. Where you store your food also plays a large part in your eating habits, bringing new meaning to "Out of sight, out of mind."

Don't worry though. There are ways to overcome these triggers.

- First, choose smaller plates to use at home. It takes less food to fill up a small plate. You're eating less, but you're still cleaning your plate and making your brain happy.

- Another way is to pre-portion your food. Have everything portioned out into single servings.

- It also helps to focus on one thing at a time. When you're eating, only concentrate on eating. Try not to watch TV or the computer while you're eating.

- Most importantly learn the true signs of hunger and avoid mindless eating. This comes in handy when you're not in control of the food.

Smoking Habits

Environmental triggers for smokers can be harder to break than triggers for overeaters. According to the American Psychological Association is in an area associated with smoking can cause a smoker to have a craving. That means they could walk into a bar where there are no cigarettes, ashtrays, or other smokers, yet still, have a craving because they associate the setting with smoking.

Your regular daily routine could also cause triggers. Some people associate their morning cup of coffee with smoking. An easy fix for that is to keep yourself busy in the morning. Try to distract yourself from the craving. You can also trade your coffee out for tea or juice.

Most smokers smoke while driving making the car another common trigger. If you have cravings whenever you drive try singing along to the radio or a CD. You could also substitute smoking with chewing gum while driving.

Stress is another major trigger for smokers. Cigarettes have thousands of chemicals in them that trick your brain into thinking that they are helping relieve your stress. The key to overcoming the stress trigger is to find new ways to relieve your stress. Meditation and yoga are both good stress management techniques.

Drinking Habits

Stress and anxiety are big triggers for drinking. As I mentioned earlier, they are also the cause for most habits.

There are two main types of triggers; external and internal. External are people, places, or things that trigger you desire to drink. They are easier to avoid than internal triggers. Internal triggers are, as the name states, inner emotions that trigger your desire to drink.

A good way to figure out exactly what causes your triggers is to track them for a week. Keep a journal with you and every time you have the urge to drink, write down what happened or where you were that caused the urge.

Some simple ways to avoid external triggers are to keep little, to no alcohol, at home. Socially, try avoiding situations that involve drinking. You may feel guilty turning down invitations to go out with your friends, but just remember it's not forever. You only have to turn them down until your urges become more manageable.

It won't be possible to stay away from all triggers. Always remind yourself why you are making this change. Keep a list somewhere on your person that you can read when you have the urge to drink. Talk to an accountability partner. That's what they're there for. Distract yourself. Find something to do to keep your mind off your urge. Lastly, you could also ride it out. Problem the hardest, but tell yourself that it's only temporary. That the feeling will pass.

Using your Triggers

You can also use your triggers for good. Task association is a good way to control your triggers. For instance, doctors have helped insomniacs by telling them to only go to bed when they are sleepy. If they can't sleep, they are told to go to a different room that way their bed is only associated with sleep. This could work to cut back on environmental triggers.

Instead of keeping snacks close to your work area, keep them in the kitchen or break room. That way you associate your desk with working and not with eating. Train yourself to associate your car with singing along with the radio instead of smoking. Only eat at the kitchen table and not on the couch. That way the couch is only for watching TV and the kitchen table is for eating.

CHAPTER FOUR

A SIMPLE BREAK

I'm going to start with the most basic three steps of breaking a bad habit. I don't want to overload you with a bunch of information. These first three basic steps will give you the building blocks to move onto more in-depth information.

The first step you have to take in breaking a habit is the decision to break the habit. You're probably thinking, "Duh," but you have to make sure you have a reason. If you don't have a reason to quit, you will not quit. You won't get anywhere if you go at this thinking you "might" have something you need to change. You have to know and want to change. Make a list of the reasons why you want to stop. If you can't think of anything, make a list of the bad things that will happen if you don't stop. For example, if you don't stop binge eating you could become overweight and develop serious health problems.

The next step is to be ready to face your boredom or emotions. As mentioned before habits are formed out of boredom or stress. You have to be willing to take a look at your life and figure out how to change what is causing your dissatisfaction. You must be ready to face the discomfort. We as humans don't like discomfort, but if you can overcome that, then you have surpassed one of the biggest hurdles. Make your life the way you want it to be.

The last step is to find a new way to relieve stress. You could have the life of your dreams, but you still suffer from stress. You feel stressed, so you turn to alcohol. You drink, and then you don't feel stressed. That makes you think you have everything together. Instead, you need to replace you drinking with something new, something healthy. You could use meditation or exercise as a healthy alternative.

The first three steps are:

1. Make sure you have a good reason to break your habit

2. Be ready to face the emotions and boredom that is causing your habit

3. Find a new way to handle your stress

Starting with these three steps will put you well on your way to breaking your bad habit. In the coming chapters, I will go into more detail on how to switch out your bad habits for new healthy habits.

A Big Break

As learned in the last chapter, there are three necessary steps to breaking habits. While those three steps are paramount there are other tips and tricks to take your habit breaking to the next level. We'll discuss several of them in this chapter, and flesh out even more throughout the rest of the book. A big part of break a bad habit is replacing it with a new one; I'll wait until later to explain how to start said new habit. Now, let's look at some tips to kick those habits to the curb.

1. Set a Start Date

Mark it on your calendar when you want to start changing your habit. You have to be serious about this, so having a countdown will help you to stay on track. The countdown will help to create excitement. Just like a child counting down the 25 to Christmas, or the days before their birthday. You want to drastically change your life for the better, so there should be an element of excitement.

2. Bait and Switch

Once you know what habit you want to change then, you can sub a new habit, temporary or permanent, in its place. If you're a nail-biter, try subbing in gum. Gum can also be used to help with smoking urges.

3. Discover your triggers

Knowing why we make certain decisions is the key to conquering your habits. Often we perform the habit without even realizing we're doing it. That's why it's called a habit. For a long time after my Dad quit smoking, every time he got in the car he would roll down the window and fiddle with his pocket because that's what he would do when he smoked. He never even realized he was doing that until we told him.

But you can fix that by being consciously aware of when you perform your habit. There are five main triggers for habits; location, time, emotional state, other people, and an immediately preceding action. Start to take notes whenever you perform the bad habit. Soon you will be able to figure out what is triggering your problem.

4. Don't go cold turkey

Everybody has probably tried to give up something cold turkey. Cold turkey is a favorite of smokers, but it rarely ever works. It's similar to telling a child to not do something, and that will be exactly what they go and do. Cold turkey is centered on perfection. People think that they if they slip up then they have failed. Nobody is perfect. Cold Turkey leaves no wiggle room, and with something like this, you need a little wiggle room.

5. Switch up your environment

You don't have to move or do anything drastic. The smallest change can switch your brain's thinking. You always smoke in the parking lot at work; the parking lot becomes a trigger. If you change your routine just slightly you will trick your brain into not craving a cigarette. You can also use the 20-second rule. Make it so that it takes 20 more seconds for you to make your habit. If you smoke, keep your cigarettes in a draw where you have to walk to get them. If you have a problem with snacking, put your snacks in the back of the pantry.

6. Make it incremental

The best way to make a change is to set daily incremental changes. You need to wean yourself off of you habit. The first step is to establish a baseline. This is going to differ according to what you want to change. Such as; how much time you watch TV, how many cigarettes you smoke each day, how many drinks you consume when out with friends. Then choose how much you're going to give up each week. If you're a smoker and you typically smoke a whole pack a day; then the first week or two you go to 15. Then the next two weeks you go down to 10, and so on until you stop smoking.

7. Don't focus on what you don't want

Most everybody that makes a goal will make this mistake. They will say, I'm not going to do this, or I'm not going to that. Setting a goal like that is setting you up for failure. Instead, decide what you are going to do. It's similar to the bait and switch. If you know you like to snack when working; instead of saying you're not going to snack, say you are going to snack on vegetables. Then all you have to do is switch your chips out for carrots.

8. Do it in honor of yourself

Research shows that people that try to break habits out of frustration or guilt will ultimately fail. People that respect themselves and are happy with who they are will be more successful. Work to change your bad habit from a position of personal strength and confidence.

9. Make a declaration

Social media has become a big part of most everybody's day. Use this to your advantage. Announce on social media the change you are going to make if you feel comfortable doing so. Then keep them updated as you progress. Chances are you will have friends that will congratulate you, and that will make you feel good about what you are doing. This one, of course, isn't for everybody. Some habits that you are trying to break may not be something you want to share with the whole world.

Some habits are very personal, so if you don't feel comfortable sharing it with a large group of people, then you don't have to. Keep in mind though having somebody to talk to can help you along the way.

10. Be prepared to forgive yourself

There will be slip-ups. We are only human beings, and we learn from out slip ups. When you slip up, forgive yourself. Wake up the next day ready to beat your habit. Don't go at it with an all or nothing attitude. There are no scorecards in life. The slip up happened, learn from it, and move on. If you are serious about beating this habit, you won't throw your hands up in defeat after a few lapses.

Classical Conditioning

Classical conditioning is a psychological learning process that occurs when two stimuli are repeatedly paired; a response that is at first elicited by the second stimulus is eventually elicited by the first stimulus alone. An example of this is Pavlov's dog.

Pavlov trained his dog to associate the thrill of being fed with the sound of a bell. He would ring a bell every time he gave the dogs their food. After several repeats of this the dog associated the sound of the bell with receiving food. The dogs would then begin to salivate every time they heard the bell.

This theory doesn't just apply to salivating dogs. Over the years it has formed an important rationale for the development, maintenance, and a relapse of bad habits.

Habits work much in the same way as Pavlov's dogs did. For a smoker, just the site of a pack of cigarettes will elicit a dopamine response causing them to have the urge to smoke. This isn't restricted to smokers either. The same dopamine response happens in alcoholics, overeaters, and so on.

This can be used in reverse, to break a habit. The bell was the trigger for the dogs to start salivating because they knew the food was coming. Just like if a smoker always lights up when they get in the car. The car is the trigger for the smoker to want to smoke. If you start ringing the bell for the dog but don't give them food they will eventually learn that the bell no longer means food. If you stop lighting up every time you get in the car eventually you won't have that trigger anymore.

This is definitely one of the more complicated and harder ways of breaking a habit, but it will work. All the rest have ways of distracting your brain, making it easier to change.

Procrastination

Everybody has been faced with procrastination at some point. It can also be detrimental in your ability to break a habit. But just like breaking a habit, you can overcome procrastination.

In a nutshell, procrastination is when you continually put off doing something. The first step, like with most things, is **realizing you are procrastinating**. If you're honest with yourself, then you know when you are procrastinating, but if you're not sure here are some ways to know;

- Waiting for the right mood, or day to start something

- Doing unimportant tasks to avoid what you need to be doing

- Sitting down to start working, then immediately going to do something else

Once you've realized you are procrastinating, then you can move onto the next step.

Figure out why you are procrastinating. It could be either you or the task. You might find the task unpleasant. Which, since you're changing a habit, you probably will find the task unpleasant. You could also be disorganized or overwhelmed. An important part of the habit breaking process is being organized and knowing what you are doing. Another reason could be that your heart is not into it. You don't have a good enough reason to change this habit.

Lastly, **adopt anti-procrastination strategies**. Procrastination itself is a habit. As you've learned, the only way of getting rid of a habit is persistently not doing the habit. The same tricks you have or will learn about breaking a habit will work to keep you from procrastination. Set up a reward system. Have somebody check in with you. Anything that will keep you accountable in some way, shape, or form.

Be Prepared

Unfortunately, a fact of the world is there will be people that want to sabotage you and your goals. It's not bad enough that you will have self-Sabotaging moments, but you will have to handle other people trying to do the same thing. You have to be prepared to ignore them. They may or may not know what they're doing. Their words can be poison to your success. The moment you start taking their words of "advice" will be your first steps towards failure. Having a plan to handle naysayers is just as important to know what you'll do when you have urges. Make sure you know what to say or do when negative comments arise.

CHAPTER FIVE

A NEW YEAR'S PROBLEM

What's something you get asked every New Year? What's your New Year's resolution? For the first few weeks of the year, every person you see will ask you the same thing. It's expected of everybody to make a New Year's resolution, yet they don't work for people. At least not the way people use them. There's a saying that the definition of insanity is doing the same over and over and again expecting a different result. Then why do people continue to try to make and keep a resolution? People think that resolutions will help them to break some of their bad habits. First, let's look at why a resolution does not work.

1. You're setting the wrong goals.

The most common resolution is to lose weight or get in shape. You wake up the first of January, hop out of bed and say, "I'm going lose 50 pounds this year." By the 15th of January, when you're supposed to be at the gym, you're watching reruns of "The Big Bang Theory" while eating a pint of rocky road. You did nothing wrong. Keeping goals takes more thought than just stating them. These types of goals have little to no leeway. When something happens, and you fail, you will be less likely to make more in the future.

2. Your resolution rarely has to do with the real problem.

You decide to run out and get that gym membership on January first. Good luck fighting the crowd. The gym is going to be packed with everybody else just like you. Once you're in there, you start comparing yourself to everybody. It will definitely help you work through deep-seated psychological issues with inadequacy, rejection, competitiveness and insecurity, but it won't help you solve the real problem. If your goal is to be healthier, then the gym might help, but if you have a problem overeating then it's not going to help. More than likely you're still coming home and eating all the calories you burned off earlier.

3. You set too many.

When making a New Year's resolution a lot of people will think, "While I'm changing this I'll go ahead a change this." Their list of resolutions ends up looking like this;

- Be a better person

- Lose weight

- Sleep more

- Learn a new language

- Drink less

And so on. I get stressed just looking at the list. Our body, as it is, is in homeostasis. It's happy and doesn't want to be changed. The brain has only a finite amount of willpower, and if you start trying to change too many things at once, the brain becomes overwhelmed. The first two weeks of keeping your 10 resolutions may go well, but then your brain starts to smoke and eventually just stops. Then you fall back into old habits.

4. They're too vague.

Let's look at the list above again.

- Be a better person

- Lose weight

- Sleep more

- Learn a new language

- Drink less

They all have something in common. They're about as clear as muddy water. There is no definite way to know if you passed or failed. It's like you teacher gave you an okay on your report card instead of an A or B.

- I want to learn a new language- Great, but what language? Are you trying to learn all languages or a specific one? How are you going to learn your new language? You have no definite plan on how to learn that mysterious new language.

- I want to lose weight- Alright, but how much? Are you overweight and you want to get to a healthier BMI? Do you just want to lose an extra five pounds to fit back into that old dress? You approach those options in very different ways. You have to know how much and why you want to lose weight.

- I want to be a better person- That's admirable, but how? How do you want to be a better person? Do you have a bad temper? Do you use your phone too much? In what way to you want to change? It's great you want to be a better person, but you have to know what aspect of you that you need to change to achieve that goal.

With this new information as to why New Year's resolutions have a tendency to fail, we can now discover how to make them work. No need to swear them off, instead learn how to make them so that you will actually keep them.

1. Be the person you want to be.

The key to keeping any goal is to imagine that you have already achieved your goal. Don't just say, "I'm going to lose weight," or, "I'm going to stop smoking." Be that person. Visualize you eating healthier and working out regularly. Everybody knows the saying "fake it till you make it," this is the same concept. The more you believe on the inside you are already there, the more it will show on the outside.

2. Make them simple.

In fact make them so stupid simple that completing one seems too easy. Remember the acronym KISS, keep it simple stupid. The simpler the goal is, the easier it is to tell that you have accomplished something.

- If you want to drink less hold yourself to drinking one less drink each day, or each week. Then the next week cut out another drink. Continue doing just that, each week, until you reach your overall goal. You'll know you're achieving your goal when you drink less this week than you did the last.

- If you want to sleep more, start setting the alarm to go to bed. If you typically go to bed at midnight, set the alarm on your phone to go off at 10:30 telling you to get ready for bed. That way you will be in bed by eleven. You'll start waking up more refreshed, and you will quickly see that you're achieving your goals.

- If you want to lose weight set your goal to eat more fruits and vegetables each week. Instead of have French fries with your burger have carrot sticks. Start switching out the high-fat sides with whole veggies. You will start seeing a significant change, and you will know you're achieving your goals.

3. Make yourself more accountable.

When people set a resolution, there's nothing that happens to them if they fail, besides the fact that they don't achieve their goal. Instead of having an easy way out, make it painful to not succeed. Dietbet.com is a website that will help you do just that. They have helped over 150,000 people achieve their weight loss goals. The way it works is you choose one of their plans, which you have to pay for. If you achieve your goal, you will win a part of the pot, the money you put in plus some. If you don't achieve your goal, you get nothing. Of course, you don't need their website to do the same thing. If your goal is to quit smoking tell everybody that if you smoke a cigarette, you will pay x amount of dollars to an acquaintance/co-worker/charity that you don't like. Not only are you giving to something or someone you don't like, but you are also spending money that you could use for something you want or need.

4. Keep the number down.

You probably have a million things you want to change, but you have to narrow down your resolution. As I mentioned before your brain only has a finite amount of change willpower. If you deplete it, then you won't achieve anything. Instead make one very simple goal, which is easy to track, and achieve that first. Once you have achieved that goal, and are confident you created a new habit, then start working on another goal.

New Year's resolutions can either help you or hurt you in your habit breaking goal. You have to be extremely careful in the execution. They can be a good way to help you achieve your goals.

CHAPTER SIX

HABIT FORMING

Bad habits. Now we're going to move into a different direction. It's easier, when trying to break a bad habit, to transform it into a good habit. Not only are you eliminating something wrong, you're also forming something good. It's a win-win. Aristotle said, "We are what we repeatedly do. Excellence then is not an act, but a habit." When you were a child learning how to tie your shoes, you had to repeatedly practice over and over again before you learned how. Now you tie your shoes without even thinking. The same goes for forming a new healthy habit.

There are a lot of programs out there that say if you do something for 21 days it will be stuck in your brain. That's true to an extent. Chances are if you have successfully done your goal for 21 days in a row; you will continue to do it. But like all things, it doesn't necessarily work for everybody or every goal. Fulfilling your goal for 21 days is a huge step in the right direction as long as you remember that you still have to actively work to maintain it.

The Three R's

I spoke earlier about the three step structure of forming a habit. You can develop a new habit using that same knowledge. The three R's are; reminder, routine, reward. 'Reminder' is the trigger for your habit. Routine is the habit itself. 'Reward' is the positive thing that makes your brain want to continue to repeat the habit.

Step one is to set a reminder for your new habit. You definitely do need motivation to start a new habit, but motivation isn't enough. And it's definitely not the only way. You have to remember to do your new habit. There are several ways to remind yourself to do something. It could simply be putting your workout clothes someplace where you will see them as soon as you wake up. Set the alarm on your phone telling you to eat a healthy lunch. No matter what it is that you want to start doing, you have to remember to do it.

Picking the right reminder is key, though. The best way I know to figure out when to set a reminder is to make a couple of lists. On the first list write down everything you do every day without fail. For example; brushing your teeth, eating breakfast, going to work, turn off lights, go to bed, and so on. Those are all good things you already do that can remind you to perform your new habit. Such as, after I eat breakfast, I'll go for a walk.

On the second list write down everything that happens to you every day. For example; you stop at a stop sign, you hear your favorite song, a commercial comes on, and you get a text. With both of this list you have a wide array of things that you already respond to that you can use as a reminder. If you want to start moving more, every time you hear your favorite song, dance to it. Don't do this if you're driving, though.

Step two is to create a habit that is super easy to start. There are lots of shows on TV showing people shedding lots of weight in a short amount of time. Or you see the runners or swimmers at the Olympics. It makes you want to achieve the same thing. Everybody has those moments where you think you can be just like them. The enthusiasm is great, but it's important to know that lasting changes are a product of habit. Remember, in the words of Leo Babauta, "Make it so easy that you can't say no." At first, performance doesn't matter. The only thing that matters is you strive to do something. Don't worry about how long you run, or how many veggies you eat, it just matters that you are running or eating vegetables. First, decide what you want your new habit to be. Then ask yourself, "How can I make this so easy that I can't say no?"

Step three is to create a reward. You have to celebrate. Celebration is an important part of life. You want to continue to do something that makes you feel good. Since you have to repeat an action for it to become a habit you have to find a way to reward yourself for doing it. If your goal is to exercise, then every time you finish a work out tell yourself, "Good job," or, "Today was a great day." You can also choose to say "Victory" or "Success" every time you practice the new habit. Give yourself credit no matter how big or small the success was.

Step by Step

That's an easy way to start adopting a new healthy habit. Some habits are going to be harder than others to adopt. Here are few other tips to help adopt a new habit.

Make the habit daily. New habits that you only do every few days are harder to adopt. If you want to start exercising, make sure you exercise once a day for the first 30 days. After the first 30 days, you can step down to three or four times a week.

Write down your goal. When you write out, with pen and paper, what you want your goal to be, it will make it seem more important. It makes your idea more real when you write it down.

Make it so you can't lose. Tell yourself you're running an experiment. You're running an experiment for 30 days by doing this new habit. Experiments can't fail. It makes it seem a lot less stressful. Nothing matters until after the first 30 days, and by that time you have adopted your new habit.

A big downfall of people adopting a new habit is that they doubt there self. When you first start working out you may have the thought, "I can't do this as well as they can." Whenever that thought pops into your head add, "But if I continue to work out I will get better at it." You can use this technique with anything.

Know what could happen. Be sure you know all the consequences of not starting your new habit, and know the impact of starting your new habit. Suppose your goal is eating healthier. If you don't start eating healthier, you could start gaining weight and develop health problems. If you do start eating healthier, you will lose weight and have more energy during the day.

Do it for yourself. Don't bog yourself down with the thoughts of what you should do. Instead, focus on what you want to do. You're making these changes for yourself and not for anybody else. Work towards things that motivate you and make your life better. Don't think you have to live your life like everybody around you does.

Switch Bad for Good

One of the best ways to break a bad habit is to switch it out for a good one. It helps to trick your brain and contributes to reduce cravings.

- As always, you have to first identify your triggers. You cannot break bad habits until you figure out what triggers them.

- For every trigger identify a good habit that you could do instead. Instead of smoking when you wake up, what are you going to do? Good habits could be; exercise, meditation, decluttering, organizing, and more.

- For, at least a month, be consistent with those triggers. Every time a trigger comes up act on the good habit you decided to do. The more consistent you are, the more the new habit will become ingrained, and the less you will think of the bad habit.

- Avoid severe trigger situations. You can't always switch out all triggers for new habits. As mentioned before, you might want to skip going out with friends after work for a little while. At least until you get a handle on controlling your urges.

- Discover ways to fight the strong urges. Even though the goal is to switch out the bad habit for a good habit, you will still get the urge to do the bad habit. You will likely need a backup plan when fighting urges.

- Find supportive help. Have somebody you can talk to if things get really rough. Some bad habits are tougher to break than others, and you will go through some tough times, so having somebody you can talk to will help you work through the tough times.

- Stay positive. There will be times when negative thoughts pop into your head. You will have self-sabotaging moments. But the key is to stay positive. When negative thoughts come up, remind yourself why you're doing this. Remind yourself that you're changing yourself for the better.

CHAPTER SEVEN

BE SUPPORTIVE

The human mind has the amazing ability to be able to talk you out of doing what you know is right. It can come up with crazy reasons why you shouldn't do something that you know you need to do. You want to work out, "Why? It will make you sweaty." You want to quit smoking, "You'll feel more stress if you do." You want to go to be earlier, "But then you'll miss Jimmy Kimmel." See what I mean. You have to find a way to tell your brain to shut up, and an accountability partner will help you do just that.

Growing up you probably had friends that you would vent to, and they would help you feel better about a situation. An accountability partner works much in the same way.

It will probably feel foreign or uncomfortable the first time. That's a good thing. The uncomfortable feeling is your brain resisting the change. Embrace those feelings. It will be worth it once you work through them.

The role of an accountability partner is to keep you accountable. They help as an outside force to tell your brain to shut up. Their only purpose is to keep you on track. They are there for you when you feel like straying from your path. They're there for you when you wake up in the middle of the night wanting a cupcake. Or when you are extremely stressed out, and you want a cigarette.

Your partner can be anybody that you resonate with. There is no need to pay a professional. They could be a family member, co-worker, friend, or somebody else that is trying to achieve the same goal. Find someone that you connect with and trust to hold you accountable. Be completely open about your goal. What you want to achieve and when you want to achieve it. They are there to be your cheerleader and to hold you to your commitment. Here are some things to look for in choosing your accountability partner:

1. They're reliable. They are easily reached whenever wherever.

2. They want to be your partner. You can't make somebody help you, so make sure they actually want to.

3. Make sure they can relate to you in some way. You don't want to pick someone that has never tried to lose weight to help you lose weight. They won't understand what you're going through.

4. You feel comfortable being honest and open with them, and they are comfortable giving you honest feedback.

Now that you know how to pick your accountability partner, let's talk about the benefits they will provide you. One of the biggest benefits to having an accountability partner is they will accelerate your performance. When you connect with someone one-on-one, you are able to work through the problems of your plan with them. You'll be able to make a sure fire plan to achieve your goals.

Your partner will help you measure your achievements. A good partner will help you to set milestones to reach along the way. It will be easier for you to keep track of your success, and keep you from becoming discouraged. Their outside eyes will see your success more easily than you will be able to.

They will help to validate your thoughts and ideas. Having someone to bounce your ideas off of, besides yourself, will help you to make decisions. They can give you honest outside information. They will help to silence your inner critic.

They help to keep you engaged. Things will come up that will try to distract you from your goals, and you will have someone there to help you stay the path. When you're bored, they will be there for you to talk to. Just knowing that you have somebody there for you will help you to keep your eye on the prize.

Ultimately they will hold you responsible. They are there behind you, pushing you towards your goals. They keep you from getting distracted and hold you accountable. Having a weekly check in with someone, and knowing you have to tell them what you have done this week to achieve your goal, will make you more likely to stay proactive. They keep you from making excuses, and, instead, make deliberate actions towards your end goal.

This isn't to say that you can't achieve your goals by yourself. There are people out there that can, but it takes a lot more willpower. Having a support system will make all the difference in the world.

CHAPTER EIGHT

BOOST YOUR POWER

And that's willpower. Willpower is probably one of the last things you need to work on though. If you don't know what you're trying to change, or why you're doing it, then willpower isn't going to help. You could have great willpower, but without a purpose it's going to fall flat. It's like building a house. You can have all the wood you need, but if you don't have the nails, it's not going to stay together. Once you have your plan in place, then you can move onto willpower.

Willpower and self-control are imperative building blocks for a happy and prosperous life. Some of the most persuasive evidence comes from these two studies.

The first is the marshmallow experiment. Psychologist Walter Mischel started the experiment in the 1960s. He would offer four-year-olds a choice of a marshmallow now or two marshmallows if they could wait 15 minutes. He and his associates then tracked those students as they grew up. They found that the children who were willing to wait 15 minutes for the marshmallows achieved greater academic success, better health, and a less likely chance of divorce.

In the second study, 1,000 children were studied from birth to 32. Researchers found that the children's self-control could predict the future of their health, substance dependence, criminal offenses, and personal finances. It was even true when they eliminated factors such as intelligence and social class.

Use it or lose it

Everybody knows these two factors about muscles:

- Muscles get stronger when exercised

- Muscles can be overworked, which leaves them weak until they have time to rest

But here are some interesting things you may not know.

- In a study, some participants were told not to think about a white bear. Thought-suppression takes a good deal of self-control, especially when told not to think about something. After that, they were told to limit their intake of beer during a taste test because there would be a driving test later. The thought-suppression participants drank more than the non-thought-suppression participants.

- In another study, participants that were asked to suppress their emotions during an upsetting movie gave up sooner during a physical stamina test than those who were freely allowed to express their emotions.

- In a third study, women watched a documentary while seated near a candy bowl. In some, the candy bowl was right next to the woman, in others the candy bowl was across the room from them. Later, they were given hard puzzles to solve. Those that had been seated close to the candy bowl gave up sooner than those who weren't.

In each of these studies, the people that were forced to overuse their willpower or self-control could not fully finish subsequent tasks. Their willpower had been depleted. Now let's look at some ways to strengthen your willpower.

1. Don't keep your willpower depleted

If you have plans to help your friend move heavy pieces of furniture, you're not going to spend 30 minutes before lifting weights. You know your energy will be depleted before you help your friend. The same goes for your willpower. Exercising self-control is an excellent way to build willpower, never giving yourself a break is a good way to deplete it.

2. Meditation

Meditation seems to come up a lot when looking for ways to change habits. It is a great way to strengthen your ability to control your thoughts. But what is meditation? Meditation is simply the practice of bringing your thoughts to the present moment. 47% of lives are spent either thinking about the past, or what has to be done in the future. Leaving us with very little time to think about what we are doing at this present moment. Our brains are very undisciplined. They like to wander. With 10 minutes of meditation each day it will help strengthen your mind and help keep it from wandering. Studies have shown after just 2 to 3 days of 10-minute meditation your brain will be able to focus better, you will have more energy and a lot less stress.

3. Use your imagination

Imagination is an amazing way to improve willpower. The body can respond the same way to an imaginary scenario as the real one. If you imagine laying on a beach, listening to the waves crash, your body will respond by relaxing. On the other hand, if you think about going to work and having a meeting with your boss, your body will tense in response. Dieters are in a constant state of depletion. As a result, they feel everything more intensely. Imagination is able to help control these irritations

In a study, participants were asked to watch a movie with a bowl of chocolate placed nearby. One group was told to imagine they had decided to eat as much as they want. The second group was told to imagine they had eaten none. The third group was told to imagine they had decided to eat the chocolate later. The first group ate more than the other two. Then when given the opportunity to eat later, those that had imagined they would eat later, ate less than the others. They even reported a lesser desire to consume the candy.

4. Use your opposite hand

Researchers have conducted studies that tested corrective actions. One they found that worked particularly well was to use your opposite hand. Your brain is wired to use your dominant hand so it will take willpower to use the non-dominate hand. To practice this, choose a time during the day to use your non-dominate hand. I would suggest doing no more than an hour at a time. More than an hour may deplete your willpower

5. Distract yourself

It's even possible to use your imagination to distract yourself from unwanted thoughts. Just like in the study mentioned earlier about the white bear. When you tell yourself not to think about something, it's going to continually pop back into your head. Train yourself to think about something else. If you don't want to think about that white bear, or cigarettes, or candy, flip your thoughts to something else. Instead of a white bear, think of a black bear. Instead of cigarettes, think of chewing gum. Instead of candy, think of fruit. That puts you in complete control of your thoughts

6. Control your stress

I have mentioned stress several times throughout this book. Stress is the main culprit of many problems. When you become stressed, you'll tend to fall back into old habits. Most of the time you won't even realize it because your body goes into autopilot. When you're stressed, your body releases stress hormones, mainly cortisol.

Cortisol increases your cravings for carbohydrates. Carbs will lower your cortisol levels. Which is probably perhaps why you turn to your friends Ben and Jerry. Alcohol is also a depressant that reduces your cortisol levels. Both of those options hold some negative side effect and aren't helping you to kick those bad habits.

Fortunately, we know these things so you can have control over what you do. The stress response is the same as the fight or flight response, so anything that counterattacks that response will do. Start responding to those stressors by listening to calming music, visualizing calming scenes, or moderate exercise. Whatever works for you. Researchers also say viewing funny videos can help counteract willpower depletion.

The more you practice these habits, the more likely they will be there to help you when major stressors arise.

7. A step at a time

Most of the time people give up on goals, not because of the lack of willpower, but because of feeling overwhelmed in what they are trying to accomplish. I have mentioned something similar to this before. Break your goals down into manageable pieces. That way you can see each step you take instead of trying to consume the whole thing. This also keeps you from depleting your willpower, keeping you recharged and ready to continue working at all times.

8. Be yourself

It takes a lot of effort to suppress you typical behaviors, personality, and preferences. Not surprisingly, it also depletes willpower. Psychologist Mark Muraven found that people who exert self-control to make others happy were more easily depleted than individuals who held true to their own goals and happiness. People pleasures may find they are at a disadvantage when it comes to willpower as opposed to those who are secure and comfortable with their self.

9. Change your speech

In another correction study, researchers conducted to modify the subject's natural speech. This would include resisting the urge to say a cuss word, or simply change from saying "hey" to "hello." It takes willpower to make the conscious effort to change one's speech, especially when we typically speak out of instinct. It doesn't matter what you do to change your speech, as long as you make a conscious effort to switch things up. Just like using your opposite hand, choose a chunk of your day where you will change the way you speak. You also need to decide what it is that you are going to change. You might choose to stop swearing, or to stop saying slang words like "ain't." Remember to only practice this for about an hour at a time, or you may deplete your willpower. After only two weeks you will see an increase in your willpower.

10. Keep temptations at bay

With most habits, you have a weakness for what you like to consume. If you drink too much keep alcohol out of your house. If you smoke, get rid of all your cigarettes. If you snack a lot, either get rid of the junk food or put it out of sight. There will be times when you see your weakness, and you will need to make a plan for that moment. Decide how you are going to handle it. If your weakness is junk food and you have children, chances are junk food is going to enter your house at some point. No matter where the kids got the food, grandma, trick or treating, school, work out a plan where you don't constantly see it. Work with your spouse or significant other. Have them take all the junk food and put it where you don't know where it is. If the kids want some, they have to ask the other parent, not you. And you have to promise that you won't beg and plead to know where it is. That takes a little willpower in itself, but a lot less than trying to keep from eating the junk food that you see.

Willpower is just like any other muscle in your body. With the right practice, it can be strengthened. I have just given you 10 ways to increase your willpower and self-control, but don't try to do all 10 at once. You'll just end up driving yourself crazy. Think of training your willpower just like you would prepare for a race. On your first day of training, you're not going to run the full 26 miles. Not unless you're already an Olympic runner. Instead, you will increase the amount you run every day. Choose one of these to start using on a daily basis. Once you feel that's not working for you anymore, pick a different one. Before you know it, you will be more mentally strong.

CHAPTER NINE

MEDITATIVE STATE

Mediation has proved to be very helpful in most aspects of life. It has shown up numerous times already in this book. Since it seems to be so useful, I figured I would dedicate a whole chapter to it. We'll take a deeper look into the benefits of meditation and how it will help you break your bad habits. Then I will give you a simple step by step on how to get started meditating for beginners. If you already meditate, then you have a leg up.

Ask anybody that meditates, and they will tell you it's good for you. But in what way? Is that just from years of practice, or is there scientific research out there that proves it's good for you? Here are some general ways that mediation can help:

- Improves willpower

- Improves focus

- Decreases stress

- Improves ability to learn

- Increases energy

There are over 3,000 scientific studies that examine the benefits of meditation. I'm going to summarize some of the findings for you.

- Decreases depression

In Belgium, a study was conducted at five middle schools involving approximately 400 students. Professor Filip Raes concluded that the students that participated in mindfulness meditation reduced indication of anxiety, stress, and depression for up to six months later. At the University of California, a similar study was conducted with formerly depressive patients and concluded that mindfulness meditation reduced ruminative thinking and dysfunctional beliefs.

- Reduces panic disorder

The American Journal of Psychiatry published a study where 22 patients diagnosed with panic disorder were submitted to 3 months of meditation and relaxation training. 20 of the 22 participants showed that their panic and anxiety had been reduced significantly, and the changes were maintained at follow-up.

- Increases concentration

Harvard neuroscientists ran an experiment where 16 people took part in an 8-week mindfulness course. They used guided meditation and integration of mindfulness in everyday activities. Sara Lazer, Ph.D., reported at the end, MRI scans showed that gray matter concentration increased in areas of the brain involved in learning, memory, emotion regulation, sense of self, and perspective.

- Increases focus in spite of distraction

Emory University did a study that demonstrated that participants with more mediation experience exhibited increased connectivity within the brain controlling attention. The neural relationships may be involved in the development of cognitive skills.

- Prevents you from falling in a multitasking trap

Multitasking is a dangerous productivity myth that will deplete you of energy and is a source of stress. Switching between tasks is costly to your brain which can cause feelings of distraction and dissatisfaction. In a study conducted by the University of Washington and the University of Arizona, human resources personnel took part in 8 weeks of in either mindfulness meditation or body relaxation techniques. They were given stressful multitasking tests before and after training. Groups that had practice meditation showed lower stress levels and a better recall of the tasks they had done. They also switched between tasks less often, concentrating on one task for a longer amount of time.

- Increases unconscious mind awareness

A study done by the University of Sussex found that people who practiced mindfulness meditation experienced a longer paused between unconscious impulses and action. They were also less susceptible to hypnosis.

- Reduces heart diseases and stroke

Cardiovascular disease kills more people in the world than anything else. A study performed in 2012, studied 200 high-risk individuals. They were asked to, either, take part in a health education class promoting better diet and exercise, or take a class on transcendental meditation. During the next five years, they found that those who took the meditation class decreased their overall risk of heart disease, stroke, and death by 48%.

- Increases compassion and decreases worry

After 9 weeks of compassion cultivation training, participants showed significant improvement in all three domains of compassion (compassion for others, receiving compassion, and self-compassion).

- Decreases emotional eating

Scientists have found that transcendental meditation decreases the likelihood of emotional eating, which helps to prevent obesity.

There is a lot more scientific information out there that proves meditation can help with all aspects of life. It's no wonder that it shows up a lot in contributing to quit bad habits.

Simple meditation practice

If you've never meditated before, I would suggest doing a guided meditation. A quick search on the internet will turn up several apps and downloads for guided meditation. Some free choices are Omvana, Headspace, Calm, Smiling Mind, and Take a Break.

If you want to meditate on your own here is a simple meditation practice designed by Headspace App founder, Andy Puddicombe:

1. Find a quiet room where you can sit comfortably upright with no distraction.

2. Set a 10-minute timer, and get comfortable in your chair.

3. Find something in your line of vision to focus on for 6 deep breaths. With each exhale, allow your body to soften as you become more relaxed. On the 6th exhale, close your eyes.

4. Focus your attention on the points of contact between your body and the chair and floor. Notice the sensation of your arms, back, and bottom on the chair, and your feet on the floor.

5. Then become aware of your surroundings. Notice all the sounds and smells around you. Anything that you can sense without your sight.

6. Then focus on your breath. Notice how your chest expands when you breathe in and how it contracts when you exhale.

7. Once you're comfortable with the rhythm of your breathing, begin to count. 1 on the inhale, 2 on the exhale, all the way up to 10. This will keep your mind focused on your breath and keep it from wandering.

8. When you make it to 10, start back over at 1. Do not count 11, 12, 13, etc.

9. While you breathe, allow your thoughts to come and go. You can't stop yourself from thinking. What you want to do is avoid lingering on one thought. The moment you realize your mind has wandered, bring it back to your breaths.

10. Continue until your timer goes off.

The first time you do this, it will probably seem awkward and weird. It's just like adopting a new habit. The more you do it, the less uncomfortable it becomes, and the easier it will be to do.

Here are some other, more advanced, mediation options:

• Candle starting

If you have problems focusing, you can light a candle and stare at it. Make sure the candle is at eye level. If you find your mind wandering, return your focus to what the flame is doing. Another level up is to stare at the candle without blinking. It will eventually make you cry which refreshes your eyes.

• Mantra

The repetition of words helps you to find calm and focus. You can find different mantras online, or you can make up your own. It doesn't matter what you say as long as it resonates with you, and you're happy with it.

- Visualization

Another fun and easy way to meditate is to visualize an idyllic being or setting in your mind. You can make it whatever you want. Embellishing it as much or as little as you need.

- Become the Observer

Become the observer of your mind. Close your eyes and focus on the spot, about an inch, above the spot between your eyebrows, third eye chakra. Begin to focus on what you mind and body is feeling, thinking and doing.

You should now be able to use meditation to help you break your bad habits, and, in the process, start a new good, habit.

I'm sure you are dying to start working on getting rid of that bad habit that's been bothering you, so I'll wrap this up. Remember to keep this simple. Don't overwhelm yourself with too many goals, or trying too many of these techniques at once. Be prepared to fail and meet naysayers, they are inevitable, but you don't have to let them control you. If nothing else, please remember you deserve to live the best life possible.

PART III

Chapter 1: Learning About Memory

The best way to improve your memory is to understand how it works.

Memory is the space in the mind where information is stored, and used from there. It can be encoded and decoded all from the one area of the brain that controls it.

Imagine that memory is a library of all the information that you have ever encountered in your life. Libraries often have rotating books. Your memory as well has rotating information. Just like libraries, the information that is rotated is based on the importance of said information.

For example, if you are not going to see a person ever again, you will only need to know their name for the duration of the conversation you are having with them, and then you don't need to remember it any further. This would use your short term memory. However, if you work with someone every day, you would need to know their name for a long amount of time. Therefore, you would commit their name to your long-term memory.

There are two forms of memory. The first form, which is called declarative, is where you physically commit something to memory. If you see something that you deem is important, you make yourself remember. Example, repeating a phone number in your head several times until you remember it.

Then there is a non-declarative memory. This is the memory you have no recollection of trying to remember. There are some things that your brain subconsciously remembers, such as street names as you pass by them.

Memory can be sometimes faulty. It is not perfect. There are lots of factors and variables that affect your memory such as the attention you provide to your different stimulus when trying to remember something and the amount of important you see on something.

Your long-term memory may fade over time if a memory has not been called upon in a while. Just as an old photograph fades, so do memories. You may find you forget how a loved one's voice sounds when they have been gone for a long time, for example.

Sensory memory

Sensory memory is a memory that is tied to your senses. Pretty much self-explanatory. However, there is more to it than that. This memory is often only committed to short term memory.

There are three types of sensory memories. There are the memories from sight, hearing, and haptic, which has to deal with touch and taste, and smell. Scientists do not know why touch, smell, and taste use the same memory functions, but they do. Hearing seems to be the most rapidly decaying in memory, while haptic seems to commit almost instantly to long term memory.

Short-term memory

Can be used alongside the term working memory. This is your memory that remembers something for a short amount of time, and then forgets it. The memories that are forgotten are often quickly are ones that are not important. Such as things you pass in a store, or someone you see on the street.

Short term memory seems to react the most to auditory stimuli. This means that when you hear something, it can be harder to forget it than when you see it.

Long-term memory

Long term memory is where you remember things for an indefinite period of time. It can decay over time. However, some things may stick with a person forever. It seems like haptic memories stay with a person the longest, even after hearing and sight memories have faded.

Long-term memory is recorded episodically and semantically, unlike the auditory fashion in which the short-term memory is recorded. This means that people may have a hard time remembering sounds over time, but they can remember things they have seen, and patterns they have noticed. Long-term memory is a bit of a mystery even to this day on how it works exactly because everyone remembers things differently.

The type of memory most people work on is their long term memory. This takes a lot of work to build up because you really cannot fight DNA. However, you can delay the onset of memory issues by strengthening your memory.

Diet

The first thing that you should work on is your diet. If you have a poor diet, then you are going to have too much fat stored in your body. Your memory relies on your body burning rather than storing fat. This is because the ketones that are created when you burn fat are essential for the creation of memory.

Ketones are pretty much brain food.

To keep ketones burning, you should try the ketogenic diet. This is where you eat fewer carbs and more fat and protein to put your body in a state of ketosis. Ketosis is where you are constantly burning ketones in your body. The ketogenic diet also helps fight Alzheimer Disease. Here is some more information about the keto diet.

What is it?

The Ketogenic diet, which is often shortened to just being called the keto diet, is a diet that is very high in fat, and low in carbs. It is proven to be a successful diet and is linked to helping prevent or even subside several health conditions, such as diabetes, epilepsy, and even Alzheimer's. This diet is used all around the world and will change what you thought you knew about carbs and fats.

This diet is obtained by drastically reducing one's carb intake. You replace the carbs that you would have eaten with fats, which makes your body focus on burning the fats that you are consuming and moving on the fats in your body. This process is known as ketosis, which puts the body into a constant fat burning state. It also burns ketones in your liver. This is how this diet combats Alzheimer's. Ketones increase brain function, and supply healthier blood to the brain, to keep the person sharp as a tack, and ready to remember, and think, about anything.

This diet also reduces blood sugar and insulin levels, so it is great if you have diabetes, or are pre-diabetic. By following this diet, if you have type two diabetes, you could actually reduce the effects of your condition, and get it under control, to the point where you may not need your medicine as often.

This diet started out in the medicinal world in the nineteen twenties. It has been around for a long time but was only recently brought to public light. It started out as an effective treatment for people with epilepsy. That's right, it began as a diet to help ease the problems from seizures, and help people control their lives. It was kind of overshadowed for a while, however, as other technologies came into play, and new medicines were introduced, but once it was determined that the medicine did not help over thirty percent of patients, the diet was reintroduced into the medical field, and brought back into popularity in helping epileptic people gain some semblance of normalcy back into their lives.

How Does It Work?

Your body needs calories to run. There are three types of calories. The calories that you get from protein, carbs, and fat. You want to make sure that you are getting most of your calories from fat. However, not just any fat. You want to get your calories from unsaturated fats, as these are the ones that burn ketones in your liver. Saturated fats are harder to burn, and do not send your body into ketosis.

You want to also make sure you are eating protein as well, as this helps your body stay strong throughout the day as it is filling as well. Without carbs, you may find that your body tries to go on a hunger strike, so make sure that you are eating plenty of protein as well. Protein also has a good fat content as well.

Keep your carbs under a hundred grams a day. A few carbs are okay, just try to eat twice as much protein and fat.

The keto diet is literally a diet in which you switch one type of calorie with another. In this case, you are switching carbs with fats, and even though it seems counter-intuitive, it is actually quite genius. You figure out how much you are consuming by counting your calories via macronutrients, which are the sections of calories that you need to have a balanced diet.

Exercise

Exercise actually helps keep your mind sharp, because it also helps you burn fat and keep your body in ketosis. You do not have to get an expensive gym membership; thirty minutes a day of light cardio should do the trick as well.

The more you exercise, however, the more fat you burn. The more fat you burn, the stronger your memory will get. The ketones you will be burning in your liver will help your brain function and keep your mind sharp.

Plus, exercise is a great time to think about things through the day. You can try to recall a memory from that day, and see how much you remember. This game is great for those who want to be able to remember their day with ease.

Reduce Stress

Have you ever been so stressed that you felt like you could not remember anything? Stress is known to affect your memory by causing you to focus only on what you are stressed about. This leads to you forgetting important things because your brain is not able to pay attention.

Play Memory Games

It may seem silly, but those matching memory games are really good for your visual memory. You know, the ones that you played as a little kid where you flipped a card over and tried to match it with another card by remembering the placement of that card? This game is good for you well into adulthood as it helps keep your memory sharp.

You can also play auditory memory games. There are several that have you listen to a sound, and then they show you something, and you have to remember the sound after seeing a picture that is unrelated to the sound. This is great for your auditory memory.

There are not many haptic memory games, however, because haptic senses are harder to create a game. Especially if the game is on a computer.

You can find a lot of these games online for free, so don't hesitate to check them out!

Chapter 2: Thinking and Problem Solving

Thought is viewed to be abstract. There is no real way to track how it works, as not everyone thinks in the same fashion. Even scans show the differences in parts of the brain that are used when thinking.

However, it is important to know how to keep your train of thought and strengthen your mind to focus better. This will be touched upon in the next chapter.

When you are thinking, it allows you to process the information you are taking in. If you were not to think, you would only act, and that could cause a lot of issues.

Psychology

Thought is designed to help people figure out what they are going to do before they try to do it. It is seen as an evolutionary aspect, as humans are the only ones to think before doing anything. Perhaps it was for species preservation, but no one truly knows. It is all theories at this point.

However, there are ways you can improve your ability to think things through if that is what you are looking to do. This is the only way that has been proven to improve your thought, and it is something that a lot of people groan about when they come across it. Problem-solving.

Use Problem Solving.

Have you ever found yourself in a difficult situation, and you are not sure where to turn? Have you found yourself wondering how to solve a certain problem? Do you often question your ability to think things through clearly? Don't fret, because you are not alone. Millions of people struggle with the ability to problem solve. However, there are ways to improve your skills.

You may be wondering what problem-solving has to do with thinking, and the answer is simple: Problem-solving forces you to use the power of thought to open your mind to the answer that may not be out in the open. By working on your problem-solving skills, you exercise your brain, which has been proven to help people think more clearly and helps them organize the thoughts that run through their mind.

Definition

Problem-solving comes with different definitions. However, at this moment, the one we will be using here is the one that is referring to common human problem-solving, not the computerized and digital problem-solving. We will define problem-solving as an act of finding out a solution to difficult, usually confusing, situations by analyzing multiple steps and by going through a process to defeat or overcome an obstacle.

Problem-solving strategies

Problem-solving, in the simplest form, is viewed as a cycle. The process goes like this: you analyze the problem, think deeply for a solution, try the solution, modify the errors, and then get the solution for the problem. And then, you have to start all over again when there is a new problem that will arise. We may not notice it, but we're doing this every day such as when deciding what to wear, searching a detour around a construction area on our way to office or work, and thinking about what we will have for lunch or dinner.

There are many different ways to look at problem-solving. If you are a math person, problem-solving probably comes to you best in mathematical form. If you are a science person, you probably approach it like the scientific method.

There is no tried and true method of improving your skills. However, there are several that are known to help, and trying them can't hurt. You are bound to find something that works for you. If you don't, that alone could be a test of your problem-solving skills, and you could try to find what works for you!

Tips for Improving Your Problem Solving Skills.

1. Dance

"There is no way dancing could in any way affect your brain." If you think this statement is true, you would be absolutely incorrect. Dancing is a great way to work on your problem-solving skills. Have you ever tried to dance? You have to coordinate each step to the beat of the music, and if you have a particularly difficult transition, then you have to figure out the best way to move through it without tripping yourself up. It is also great exercise, which is good for the brain.

Dancing burns ketones in your liver, which functions as food for your brain. This will help you brainstorm like a pro, and really get to show off what that brain of yours can do.

2. Work out Your Brain

"Logic games are for children. Adults are too old to play silly games." Another incorrect statement. Logic games stimulate your brain and help exercise it. You see, your brain is a muscle as well as an organ, and if you do not exercise it, it begins to get weak. Logic games help keep your mind sharp, and they can be fun as well. There is nothing childish about being on top of your mental strength.

It is important to exercise your brain, along with your body to really give yourself the best chance at having a strong mind to amp up your thought processes.

3. Put on the Tunes and Move

"Music is a distraction, and will get in the way." Look at us, clearing up misconceptions one myth at a time. It is actually scientifically proven that music helps stimulate brain function. That coupled with exercise is a double threat and thinking about a difficult problem to make it a triple threat.

Although physical workouts can help you think more focused and get your blood flowing to your brain, it still does not necessarily help you solve a problem, nor it improves your skills in problem-solving. However, when you add music to your exercise, you add another thing in the background which forces your mind to focus more. Thus, music can help you increase and improve your problem-solving skills significantly.

Even if you are not working out, put on some music and try to do some logic puzzles. The music will pull your mind in a different direction, making it harder for you to concentrate, thus strengthening your problem-solving skills that much more efficiently.

4. Keeping a journal

"Only teenage girls keep journals." Misconceptions everywhere. The truth is, some of the most renowned scientists and intellectuals keep journals in order to organize their often eccentric thoughts. It is impossible to remember every fleeting thought that passes through your mind, but if you write them down, you don't have to.

Journals are great for brainstorming as well. You can jot down all of your ideas that you are having and be able to pick the best one by comparing them. This is a great problem-solving tool.

6. Distance yourself from the problem

"If I am distant from a problem, it will be harder to solve." This is the opposite of correct. When you are too close to a problem, you create a barrier between the solution and your own mind. You have to take a step back so you can look at it from all angles.

It can be hard to look at a personal problem objectively. However, if you get too caught up in the problem, it can make it harder to find the best solution, because you will be biased about what to do or say to get the problem fixed. While in the long run, you may fix the problem, you can overlook a smarter and more efficient way to finish it up.

Chapter 3: Learning and Attention Performance

You know the phrase "you learn something new every day"? It is honestly true. Every day you take in new information, and that is exactly what learning is. Learning is the act of taking in information that has already been processed. You can learn through play, teaching or rote. However, teaching is actually the least effective way to learn. Many people have to experience the information first hand.

People learn in a way that is far different than animals do. While animals learn from extensive training, human learn mostly through education. Someone would teach them what he or she needs to know. Commonly, learning occurs outside the comfort of the home.

Rote learning

One of the most common ways that humans learn is through rote learning. This is the act of memorizing something. There is a special way you go about memorizing the information though. You have to write it down, say it, and see the information. The idea is that the more you handle the information, the more you will remember.

Not everyone learns the same way, which makes it difficult to pinpoint a specific way to help you learn with ease. However, improving your attention span will help increase your learning abilities a bit, as you will be able to focus more on the information you are learning.

A lot of people have a hard time focusing, so they find that they have to work harder to get their work done. However, there are ways to improve your attention span and focus, and here are some tips.

How to Improve Your Attention Span and Focus

Many people struggle day in and day out with being able to focus on their daily tasks properly. If you are one of these people, you are not alone, and there are other people in the world who are going through the same problem. In fact, over eighty percent of the world's population has trouble concentrating from time to time in varying degrees.

Some people have problems focusing daily, while others tend only to have problems if they have a lot on their plates. No matter the reason, you can beat the distractions and regain laser-like focus just by knowing how it works, and have some tips on how to keep yourself on track.

Environment

If you are in an office space. Chances are your surroundings are very boring. Some people can work well in boring scenery, and others need something to break the monotony to keep their mind from wandering. Even if you can work in a boring workstation, personalizing your space a bit may boost your morale on days where you are a little stressed, thus allowing you to leave your stress behind and work harder and focus better.

ꓥ
Be comfortable: If you need to bring in your own office chair, do so. Comfort is the number one contributor and detractor for focus. You have to be comfortable so that you do not constantly have to break concentration to move around. If you are comfortable, you will be able to focus well, as you do not have to move at all.

ꓥ
Add pictures: Pictures can break up the monotony of your boring space. If you are a college student, your desk is probably where you spend your life learning, so why not adorn the walls around it with some motivational landscapes or some pictures of things you enjoy. This will

break the monotony and give you something to look at to keep your mind from wandering. Just stay away from pictures that have words as those can be distracting.

A

Detour the noise: earplugs, earphones, and other sound canceling objects are a gift from heaven. These things keep you concentrating on your work, rather than the world around you. If you are in a noisy environment, try putting on some headphones and playing some classical music to drown out the world around you. Classical music is great to help you learn because it opens your mind. Try it out sometime.

Nutrition

The famous mantra says you are what you eat. What you put into your digestive system will affect your ability to focus. Your diet plays a huge role in your brain's functionality. If your brain does not receive the proper nutrition it needs, then it will not function properly as it should.

A

Drink water: Your brain needs you to stay hydrated in order for it to properly function. If you are dehydrated, it makes it harder for you to focus, because your brain is starting to shut down to preserve itself. If you don't drink enough water, it is equivalent to literally drying out your brain. If you don't think that sounds scary, I am not sure what would scare you.

Eat breakfast: Have you ever been really hungry? Did it make you have a hard time focusing? Hunger is one of the largest focus detractors there are. Your body needs food to function, and as a defense, when you get to a certain point food becomes all you can think about. It is best to start your day off right with a balanced breakfast so your body can make it to lunch and your mind can stay on track.

Get up and move around: Digestion of food can be an uncomfortable process, so don't be afraid to aid it by moving. This will also help get more blood flowing to your brain. While moving around too much can distract you, taking a quick walk will help you get your mind clear and ready to learn.

Mindset

Mind over matter is another way to handle focus difficulties. Even if you have a problem with concentrating due to a disorder, you can still improve your focus by taking control of your mind. This will allow you to focus more than you ever thought was possible.

⚓ *Set aside time to deal with worries*: Worrying and anxiety is the number one killer of productivity. Worrying too much can kill your thoughts throughout the day, making focusing tedious and wearisome. Later in this book, we will learn how to balance work and homelife that will help you focus better.

⚓ *Focus on one task at a time*: This may seem to go against everything that you know. However, the truth is, it is harder to learn when you are multitasking. This is because your focus is divided amongst different things, and you cannot truly give your undivided attention to what you need to be focusing on primarily. Focusing on one task at a time will help you absorb more information from the subjects you are trying to learn.

⚓ *Close your email box and chat program*: When you are trying to learn new material, it can be tempting to take that time to also answer messages from people you know. However, that detracts from the time you have to learn what you are trying to learn. Shut down the phone, and turn off your notifications on your laptop. Just focus on the task at hand. If you take the time to really focus on what you are learning, you will find you absorb so much more information.

Prioritize: Not know what to do next can kill your focus because it will eat your time figuring out what task to do next. It will stress your brain to remember things that you should not miss or forget. To avoid this, spend a little time in the morning to plan ahead your day. Make a list of what needs to prioritize and how to finish each task.

Switch between high- and low-priority tasks: Many people prioritize their tasks at work from high to low. They work on the more important projects and leave the low-priority projects for last. This might seem effective for some people, but it can actually bog you down causing your brain to lose focus when starting to work on the projects that have low importance. By alternating high and low tasks, you give your brain a break making you focus longer. Thus, it will allow you to finish tasks in less time.

More Tips for Improving Your Concentration

🜊

Take short breaks: Have you ever had cram session, and then found that you couldn't remember a thing you read. This is actually a pretty common occurrence. Your brain needs time to rest. Just like with a machine, sometimes you have to give it time to cool down. They can't run 24/7. You are only human. Give yourself a schedule where you study for an hour and take a five to ten-minute break. This will allow your brain to rest and reset so you can retain more information.

🜊

Do your hardest tasks when you're most alert: Don't save that cram session for last minute before the big test. Do your bulk studying after breakfast. This is when your brain is typically the most alert, and you have the best chance to remember everything you studied. Saving these study sessions for when you are so tired all you can think about is sleep will kill your memory and make it harder to learn.

🜊

Look busy: Find something that will make you look busy. Perhaps put a do not disturb sign up or wear a phone headset. This way people will know not to disturb you. If you look like you are busy, many people will wait until you are not busy to ask you a question, which allows you to learn in peace.

⚹

Promise yourself a reward: Self-rewards is a great way to stay motivated to focus. It can be simple such as work for an hour and get a snack from the vending machine if you are successful. The trick is to hold yourself accountable if you do not meet your goal. No goal, no reward.

⚹

Schedule email downloads: The reality is, emails do come in, for unknown reasons, at the most inconvenient times. This may be common, but it can actually distract your focus especially when you get tempted to check the emails constantly. If so, you should set a time within your day to answer emails. Once you set on a specific schedule, train yourself to download emails only at that specific period of time.

Think of Your Mind as a Muscle

Your mind is not just a typical body organ. It is also a working muscle, an essential one. It can work with heavy workloads just as how your arms and back can, except your mind works mentally rather than physically.

What do you think would happen if you did not exercise your brain? If you think nothing would change, that is where you are wrong. Many people have the misconception that their brain will function the same forever, and that is why dementia and Alzheimer's are so devastating and tragic in our eyes. You see it as an unavoidable tragedy, but the truth is, they can be avoided if you treat your mind like a muscle. Work it out, and feed it the right nutrition.

Think of your day as a workout for your brain. Do you go to the gym every day and just focus on your chest? No. You most likely rotate your exercises in a pattern so that every part of your body gets a workout. You should do the same with your mind. Find different exercises for your brain and cycle through them.

Just as how you can hit a wall with a workout, so you can with your concentration. When hitting this wall, you simply have to dig a deeper to sought the motivation that will push through. A promise of reward can help. Nevertheless, working hard will strengthen your brain – your memory. Here are some useful tips that will definitely help you do just that:

Fighting for Attention

Technology can both save and destroy our attention spans. While there are apps you can use that silence your phone during times where you need to focus, a lot of people do not have the will power to do so with vigor. Many people will find themselves turning off this app and going back to using their phones and being distracted.

Humans are easily distracted creatures. That is why robots are so popular. They can do twice the work most humans can because they do not get distracted. As a whole, the human race could seriously use some work on their attention skills.

Of course, if you are reading this, you probably want to improve all of your cognitive skills. Whether it may be to combat the robots, or just to get through the work day, it is good that you want to fight the technology blues and get back to a strong mind.

One of the easiest ways to get a strong attention span is to go zen. Zen is where you get so lost in your work that you forget the world around you even exists. This is a wonderful thing because when you are in that state, you forget your troubles and your worries. It may seem a little strange that you want to get lost in your work that much, but it can make the time go faster, and you can learn so much more because at that moment it is just you and your information.

Meditation is a great way to help yourself achieve a zen state of mind. Meditation involves getting out of your body and into your mind. You do not have to sit cross legged and mutter "hmmm, " but you do have to be comfortable enough to let your body move over so you can enter your own brain.

When you meditate, you will have a moment where it seems like everything on your body itches. You will have the urge to scratch everywhere. Your body likes to be the center of attention. Ignore it, and it will grudgingly allow your mind to take over. Once you are in this state, you can focus more clearly on your work. From there you will find the clarity of mind that you have is out of this world, and you will learn so much more.

Everyone faces the struggle of maintaining focus. That is normal and is something that you should not be ashamed of. However, if it regularly causes you delay with your work, then you should probably strive to become better at focusing. This chapter contains a bunch of tips that will help you do so. These tips are even more perfect for people who struggle with attention deficiency.

Everyone struggles from time to time when it comes to

maintaining focus. That is nothing to be ashamed of. However, if it regularly impedes with your work, then you should strive to become better at focusing. This entire chapter is filled with tips on how to do so, and here are even more. These tips are for people who struggle with attention deficiency.

PART IV

Chapter 1: Different Emotions and How to Handle Them

There are many different emotions that a person experiences and each one of these emotions can have a range of facets that make what each person feels a wholly unique experience. This means that what you experience when you meet a new person will be entirely different from the experience you would get from anyone else. Every person is a different feeling when you first meet them, and this is a great way to learn to distinguish whose feelings you are feeling, even when you cannot experience them.

However, to be able to distinguish a person from the emotional identification card they leave, you must first be able to first understand the different emotions and be able to distinguish them from the other emotions in the atmosphere. You also have to learn how to harness them for yourself, and really get in tune with them Then, eventually, you will be able to identify someone by the emotions they leave behind. This chapter will inform you of the different emotions, and how you can understand them better.

Happiness

Happiness is a common emotion for people to experience, however, it has many different factors in it. There are several layers of happiness, and you have to be able to discern each one from the next. Being able to do this is one of the most difficult things an emotional master does because happiness is one of the most complex emotion a person feels.

Think of the best thing in your life. How it made you feel. Now think of the day you got some good news. The happiness you experienced in those two events was probably exponentially different. This is how happiness works. You can be mildly happy, or you can be happy while sad at the same time, or you can be extremely happy. There are so many different types of happiness that it can make your head spin. For this book, we will focus on the main types of happiness, so as not to cause information overload. Here are the main types of happiness.

Joy

This is the emotion that many people experience when they hear good news. It is the emotion you experience when you find out someone you know is going to have a baby. It is the basis for all happy moments. Joy is the emotion you feel when you wake up on a Saturday morning and realize that you do not have to go to work that day, and can sleep in an extra hour. Joy is the emotion you feel when you find out that you have a little more money in the bank than you originally thought.

This is the most common happiness that people feel. It can be strong, or it can be mild. It can hit all at once, or it can build gradually. Joy is everywhere around you. People often mistake joy for other emotions of happiness, however, believing that they are synonymous. They might be in the English language, but they are not synonymous in the emotional IQ culture. Each emotion is separate, not all considered one. Joy is the basic emotion of happiness, but it is not the only one.

Elation

Elation is another facet of the emotion of happiness. Elation is what you experience when you find out you got the job promotion that you have been wanting for so long. Elation is the emotion that people who have been waiting years to conceive experience when they find out that they are expecting a baby. Elation is the purest level of happiness. It leaves the person experiencing it feeling like they are on cloud nine, and like they have never felt anything better. This is the emotion of happiness that everyone seeks out and wants to experience on a regular basis.

Most people experience elation the best when they have been through a period of sadness. The sadness allows them to truly appreciate the happiness that has been bestowed upon them. When people feel truly elated, it is because something that they have wanted to happen for a long time finally happened after a long period of struggling.

Excitement

Most people know what excitement is. It is the emotion you experience when you are wanting something, and you know that it is coming, and you are so happy that you cannot wait for it to be here. Like a kid on Christmas, or an expectant mother, to someone waiting for a package in the mail. You cannot beat the feeling of excitement. It is the most contagious of emotions that are out there. When someone sees that another person is excited, they get excited for them, just so they can feel excited too.

Most people want to feel excited about each day as they wake up, however, this is nearly impossible to achieve. They can, however, achieve the next emotion of happiness that is on our list.

General Contentment

This is the last emotion of happiness that is on the list. This is what most people strive for in their life. While most people want to experience excitement every day, they are generally willing to settle for general contentment. That is because general contentment is a great feeling to have. It is when you wake up every day thinking that it is going to be a good day, and you are generally pleased with the day's occurrences. People who experience general contentment are happier people, and they are the ones you see who think that life is great.

There are a lot of people that try to fake general contentment when in reality they are not happy at all. However, since you are reading this book, you can probably already spot those people from a mile away. The people with true general contentment are the ones that you can feel the calm rolling off of them. They are the roll with the punches kind of people that you see that never have a bad thing to say about the day no matter what day you see them. Even on Mondays.

Those are the main facets of the emotion happiness. There are more subtle ones, but you could write an entire book on all the subtle nuances of happiness, and for a beginner, that is a lot of information to process in one sitting. These ones are the ones that you will experience most in the beginning. However, there are many places that you can research online to learn more about this emotion when you are ready.

Sadness

Sadness is an emotion a lot of people face. It is pretty complex as well, just like with happiness. However, it does not have as many facets, just different levels of sadness. These levels do not really have names, and they are hard to identify as anything other than sadness. The difference is when someone is depressed, as opposed to sad. With depression, not only is the sadness overwhelming, the complete apathy for everything that rolls off of them is scary. Yet, when you look at the faces of these people, they seem like the happiest people on earth.

Sadness is not depression, though. Sadness is just an emotion that you experience when something that is upsetting happens. You can experience sadness when you do not get something right, or do not get what you want. These are a few of the more general types of sadness. The slightly dark feeling you get when you are upset.

Sadness can also raise in intensity. The feeling of sadness you get after a bad break up, for example. The cliché is that the woman sits on her couch watching chick flicks while eating ice cream straight from the tub, and the guy goes out to the bar to drink away the pain. However, many people cope with sadness differently. Some may stay in bed until they feel better, some may go for a run to make themselves feel better.

Sadness can increase in intensity even more than the pain you feel during a breakup. The sadness you feel when tragedy strikes. Such as losing a loved one or a pet. This sadness can easily turn into depression if not addressed soon enough. This level of sadness often feels like a hole has been ripped in your chest. Like you could never breathe again. This is the worst type of sadness, and the hardest to get through, but if someone can get through it, they may be able to escape the grasp of depression.

Anger

Anger is one of the least complex emotions you will experience. It is pretty straightforward. However, it is also the hardest emotion to describe. Anger is like a searing branding iron is trying to rip its way out of your soul through your stomach. It leaves you feeling like you want to scream, or punch someone, or curse up a storm. I think the reason that anger is so hard to explain is that everyone experienced it so differently. It may not be very complex in that it doesn't have a lot of levels or facets, but it is experienced differently by person to person. More so than any other emotion out there. Anger can cause a wash of sadness over some people. Some people when they are angry feel strangely happy. Some people respond with mild anger on intense things, but rage on little things. It is all dependent on the person themselves, and that is why anger can be one of the hardest things to explain.

Anger can be found in many places. Most of the time it is when someone is mean to another person, however, some people respond to sad things with anger. Anger is often used as a synonym for frustration, but this is not the case. Far from it, actually. Frustration is just mild irritation at a slight annoyance. Anger is the feeling of great agitation at things that are considered harmful or offensive.

Jealousy

This is an emotion that everyone will experience in their lifetime, but no one will want to admit it. That is because, in a lot of religions, it is considered a sin. This one is one of the most hidden emotions, but one of the easiest to feel once you are tuned into it. Jealousy is the emotion that people experience when they want something that someone else has. Jealousy is also used to describe how a woman or man feels in a relationship. Do not confuse this, as it is not truly jealousy. Jealousy is when you want something that is not yours. When you already have something, and you want to protect it, that is being territorial.

Jealousy is often felt with a sick feeling in the stomach and is portrayed as a puke green aura. Have you ever heard the phrases "green with envy" or "sick with jealousy"? These are because that is the energy that this emotion gives off, and can really affect an emotional master because it is a strong emotion, due to the fact that it is generally buried deep beneath the surface, and it builds pressure until it is to the point where if it were a gas, it would cause the person feeling this emotion to literally explode.

Those are the different emotions that people experience on a regular, or semi-regular basis. Now that you know them, and their basic identifiers, you can move on to how to harness their usage to handle a situation.

Chapter 2: Meditation for Emotion

There are many ways to unlock your emotional IQ and really access it, but meditation is the best way to do so. It allows you to center yourself enough to make sure that you are finding the right part of yourself to unlock. A lot of times even if you do not do it right, you can trick yourself into thinking that you have, and you will feel like you are seeing the world when really it is a placebo effect and you are just as blind as you were before. So meditation is a great choice, though other choices will be discussed in a later chapter just to cover all options.

What is Meditation?

Meditation is the act of calming yourself and slowing your breathing to truly find your center. It is used by people from all walks of life, though it is mainly attributed to being used by monks to find inner peace. However, anyone can meditate and find it effective. You do not have to be an expert either. There are so many tutorials out there. This chapter will cover meditation techniques as well, to ensure that you are learning everything you need to know about opening your emotional IQ. You want to open it to find yourself, and meditation will help with that.

Meditation involves being able to sit still for long periods of time, so it can be difficult at first. Even more so if you are someone who is always moving, and never slows down. Because you have to slow down for meditation to even work. When you are meditating, you are literally putting

144

yourself into a trance, and your heart will slow to the pace that it functions at when you are asleep.

Meditation is used to find spirituality, along with a whole list of other things, including the emotional IQ. Here is a list of things that meditation helps with.

- ☐ Anxiety: Anxiety is a problem that plagues a lot of people. It causes raised heart rate, intense and sometimes borderline asthmatic breathing problems, and thoughts that can be suicidal, or homicidal. Anxiety attacks can leave the person who suffers from them emotionally and physically exhausted. Anxiety is also something that can be almost entirely cured my meditation

- ☐

The reason for that is when you meditate you calm yourself enough to figure out what is causing your anxiety so you can address and fix the problem. You want to be able to do that when it comes to your inner eye so that your vision is not clouded by your fears and panic attacks.

- ☐ Stress: Stress can cause a lot of problems in your life. It is the number one cause of heart attacks due to the fact that it can raise your blood pressure. It can also cause strokes and other health issues. You do not want to die due to stress as it is not a pleasant way to go.

Meditation helps you slow your heart rate and work through the things that are bothering you to ensure that you are living a healthy lifestyle. You want to be healthy, otherwise, you will find that your life will not be as enjoyable as you would hope. You want to enjoy your life. Stress can also cloud your emotional IQ just as anxiety does, and it can cause anxiety as well. You want to have a freed up emotional IQ so that you can find yourself.

- Ease Pain: By slowing your heart and breath rate, you are dulling the nerve endings in your body, allowing the pain receptors to have a break. This helps you recover from severe pain, and end chronic pain. Pain can affect your everyday life in ways that some people can never imagine. It leaves you tired, drained, and wondering where you are going to get the energy to even eat.

You do not want to live with chronic pain, but unfortunately, some people have no choice. If you meditate, however, you will be able to ease your pain for a while in order to get your energy back so that you can take on the world. This is a good thing because pain can cloud your mind, not just your emotional IQ, but your entire mind.

☐ Calm Your Soul: This is a good thing that you can use meditation for. If anything is bothering you, you can use meditation to really figure out what exactly is nagging at the back of your mind. You want to have a clear head when you go to use your emotional IQ, otherwise, you will find that what is bothering you will make its way into your sight and cause you to have some issues deciphering what is real and what is fabricated by your emotions.

It is important to separate your emotions from your emotional IQ because you have to stay completely neutral on any topic you are looking for clarity on. Otherwise, your "vision" may be skewed in the direction of your worry. You do not want that to happen, as it can cause unnecessary stress, which as mentioned above is bad for your health.

☐ Stabilize Your Life: It is important to stabilize your life because maintaining balance is essential to succeed in your life. If you do not have balance, you will have problems keeping an organized life. Having a clear and stable life is good for your health as well because you are more likely to make healthier choices. This will extend your life and make it easier to access your emotional IQ. It is proven that the healthier you are, the easier it is to clear your mind.

There are many other things that meditation can do for some people that it cannot do for others. It is best to try it for yourself to see if it works for you. Of course, if you do not know how to meditate, it can make it harder to do so, so let us go over how to meditate successfully.

How to Meditate

There are many different ways to meditate, but meditation is important to do correctly, otherwise, you will find yourself not getting the full benefits of the process, as you would if you do it correctly. So for a beginner, it is best to not take any shortcuts and to really go the full nine yards to do it correctly.

It will take some time to really learn how to clear your mind, so if you do not get it on the first try, do not get discouraged. No one gets it on the first try, and that can get frustrating, but it is completely normal. You want to keep trying to clear your mind. If you get discouraged after the first try, you won't be able to truly know if you can do it or not. Media portrays meditation as something you can do with ease and something that everyone is able to just sit and do, but it is not. It takes a lot of self-restraint. So let's go over the steps.

- ☐ Step One: The first step is to find a quiet place where you will not be interrupted. Even if it means going into the bathroom and turning the shower on to find some peace and quiet. You have to be quiet and undisturbed in order to find your inner peace. If you are not in a peaceful area, finding your center will be extremely hard because there will be so many distractions in the area that you will not be able to concentrate on yourself.

Step Two: Sit in a comfortable position. A lot of people choose the crossed leg style because that is what they know, but if it is not a comfortable position for you, then you will not be able to focus on yourself because you will be too distracted by your leg going numb, your back hurting, your hips getting stiff. If you cannot focus on anything other than your discomfort, then you are not going to be able to successfully meditate. So find the most comfortable sitting position for you, even if it means in a chair. However, do not lay down. It is too easy to fall asleep if you are laying down, because your body equates the slow heartbeat and breathing with sleep, and your brain will begin to slow as well. You want the health benefits of sleeping with the full mental capabilities of being awake. Otherwise, you will not be able to probe your mind the way you would when sitting. How you sit does not matter, as long as you are comfortable.

Step Three: Focus on your breathing. Most people say to focus on your heart rate at first, but that is a lot harder, and if you slow your breathing, generally your heart will follow suit. You want to really focus on your breath though. Do not let yourself get distracted.

Breathe in for four counts and out for four counts. Balance is key. In fact, why don't you give it a try right now? You don't have to try to meditate, just work on the breathing.

Sit comfortably, and close your eyes. Breathe in for four counts through your nose. Hold it for two counts, and then let it out of your mouth for four seconds. Focus on keeping a steady rhythm. If you lose count, then start again. You have to make sure that you are keeping the rhythm and not losing count, otherwise, you will not be able to focus on the meditation if you can't keep your breathing steady. Try doing a repetition of ten, and once you get that down, try upping it to twenty, and so on and so forth. The longer you can go while focusing on your breathing, the easier it will be to transition your focus to your mental state once you get to that point.

☐ Step Four: Ignore the twinges. This is something that is one of the hardest things to do when you are trying to get into meditation because our bodies are not meant to sit still for extended periods of time. After five to ten minutes of sitting still, you will begin to feel itchy in places such as your nose or your head. Maybe your leg will start to feel like it is going to fall asleep. Ignore all of these. They are signals from your brain to your body checking to see if you are asleep yet or not. Once the brain realizes that the body is not responding, then it will command the body to shut down all processes as if you were asleep. If you are still awake, you will get all of the benefits of being asleep, while still getting to enjoy the benefits of being awake in a calm, unfazed perception.

Step Five: Once you get into this phase of pretty much lucid dreaming, slowly transition your focus from your breathing to your mind. Do this by only focusing on every other count and when you are not focusing on your count, then focus on a thought that has been on your mind all day. Eventually, you can switch your focus entirely to that thought. Once you are ready to move on you can think of other thoughts slowly until you are fully immersed in your own mind.

Step Six: Explore your mind freely. Get to know every little nook and cranny of your brain. This step will take some time to get to, as you will need to be able to hold the meditation stage for quite a while before you can freely explore your mind. However, once you get to this stage, you will be able to learn more about yourself than you probably ever wanted to know. This is important because you want to know everything about yourself. This includes the good, bad, and even the ugly. The more you know, the more clear your vision can be.

Step Seven: This is the final step of meditation, known as the outro. A lot of people think that you can just snap out of a meditation, and some people can, although it is not very healthy for you because the sudden return of a normal heart rate stresses your heart out, and it can cause some severe headaches as well. You have to gradually enter yourself back into reality. If you do not, you will have a problem with being confused, headaches, and much more. To come back to reality without these problems, simply revert your focus slowly back onto your breathing, and focus on speeding up your breathing until your heart rate returns to normal.

Once you have successfully managed to meditate for the first time, you will find that every time after that you can begin to get a little faster with your meditation. This is a good thing because when you meditate, sometimes you do not have a lot of time, however, you still have to ease out of it. So it is good to be able to get quick at it in order to have ample time to ease out of it.

Remember, the first several times it can be extremely difficult for you to get into a trance state if you even manage to at all. Do not get discouraged if you cannot do it immediately. Also, even if you do get into a trance state it may be hard for you to maintain it for any length of time. This is normal and is nothing to feel bad about. Keep trying, and eventually, you will be able to meditate like a Tibetan Monk.

Chapter 3: Self-Discipline

It is important for you to have self-discipline when you want to improve your emotional IQ. It will help you harness your emotions exponentially so that you can work on keeping them under control. Here is how you can do that.

About Improving Self Discipline

You are probably aware that self-discipline is a great trait to have, and maybe you are not as disciplined as you should be. If that is the case, you may find it hard to keep your mind and emotions in check. If you are not able to control your emotions, your emotional IQ will be way below what it should be.

To truly understand self-discipline, you must first know the definition of what it is.

Self-discipline is defined as the ability to find a reason to stick with something for a long period of time, even if you may not want to. Especially if you do not want to.

This may seem confusing because it doesn't seem possible to find a reason to do something when you obviously do not want to do it. However, the truth is that there are reasons you may never have even known about to do what you do not want to do. Most of those come from inside yourself. The biggest reason should be for your emotional health. The more it wears down, the less you understand your own emotions.

Why You Should Improve

Do you have days where you just feel worn out? Maybe not even just physically, but mentally and emotionally as well? Do those days seem to be more often than not? If this is the case, you need to work on handling your emotions with more strength and understanding.

The reason you feel so drained is that you are letting yourself get too emotionally worked up by little things. It is human nature to get upset easily it seems. However, with a little effort in the discipline area, you can increase your emotional strength and intelligence quite a bit. This will help you find the strength to ignore the irritating things and live a happier life.

What it Takes to Develop Self-Discipline

No one is born with innate amounts of self-discipline. We are all born with a need to take care of, rather than a need to take care of others. That is why babies are not born able to walk. You have to develop yourself discipline beyond what you may naturally develop growing up.

Most people need a few things to happen to be able to work on their self-discipline, and that is okay because developing self-discipline in itself takes a form of discipline that not everyone is used to.

You have to know how to build your self-discipline though, as it does not happen overnight. You should also remember that you have taken years to be who you are, and you should not expect to change completely in a short amount of time. You have to give yourself the time to really become a better, more disciplined person. One of the hardest things about having self-discipline is developing it, and a lot of people give up before they hit their goal. So always remember to never give up, and to follow these tips to help you out.

Keeping Yourself Accountable

You are responsible for your own emotions. You cannot hold someone else responsible for how you feel, even if they make you feel that way. You can ask them to apologize for upsetting you, but in the end, it is up to you to feel better. Wallowing in your self-pity, and holding a grudge shows a low emotional IQ, and is what you want to work to stay away from. At the end of the day, you should be able to let go of everything that is bothering you and set yourself free from the chains of negativity.

Having Rewards and Penalties

Just like when you were a child, you should reward yourself for the good, and penalize yourself for the bad. Remember, you have to hold yourself accountable, and this means to only reward yourself for a good job. If you go a day without letting negativity bother you, or getting emotionally overstimulated from a minor transgression, buy yourself an ice cream cone. If you did happen to let your emotions control you, you don't get the ice cream cone. Of course the reward doesn't have to be ice cream, that is merely an example of how you should handle the situations.

The reason you should have a rewards system is that it helps you hold yourself accountable. If you had no rewards coming for a job well done, would you be just as eager to do the job right? Most people would not. It helps give you a reason to get better and to discipline yourself.

Rewarding yourself for a job well done also helps you see how far you have come based on a number of times you have been able to reward yourself. This will keep you from being discouraged, and feel like you are making no progress. Remember, staying on the track to being self-disciplined is a discipline all on its own.

Make a Commitment

You have to be committed to your goal if you want to get yourself where you want to go. You can't just make a goal with the attitude "If I don't get there, oh well.". You have to make a goal with an "I will do whatever it takes to make that goal" attitude. This is how you go from just a person with a goal, to a person who is going to make a change.

When you make a commitment to be stronger with your emotions, you are making a commitment to having a happier, healthier life. If you want to feel free from emotional chains you have to be more self-disciplined, and not let anyone control your emotions, or let your emotions control you. You have to make a commitment to being in control of your emotions. Without that commitment, you are likely to fall back into your old ways. No one wants to see you fail, and you should not want to see yourself fail. When you make that commitment, make it with every fiber of your being.

It doesn't matter if you tell the world about your goal, or if you keep it to yourself. All that matters is that you make that goal, and you commit to following through with every aspect that will get you to that goal.